FROM DEATH TO LIFE

How One Organ Donor Saved the Lives of Two Friends

TIM HAWKINS

WITH INTRODUCTIONS BY

Fred Nelis and Gordon Veldman

To an anonymous thirty-two-year-old donor, who made the ultimate sacrifice, and to the generous decision of his family to see beyond their grief to save the lives of complete strangers. Without that decision, there would be no story to tell.

Acknowledgments

The author wishes to acknowledge the contribution of Mary Beth Crain, whose early research and initial drafts of several chapters helped this important story to be told.

The author also thanks those readers who reviewed early drafts of the manuscript and provided valuable, critical insight. These include: Lou Blouw, Prof. Cliff Christians, Priscilla Christians, Jane Hawkins, Brad Heavner, Steve Kitsch, Dr. Don Knoechel, Dr. David Langholtz, Ilsy Murillo, Jean Nelis, Dick Tupper, Dr. Steve Van Wylen, John Vande Bunte, Rob Vensas, Kathy Vogelsang, Dr. David Young, and Nancy Zielinski.

This is the true story of two friends—
a swimmer and a sailor—
and how they became
the "Transplant Brothers."

Contents

SECTION ONE

The Transplant Brothers

How the Lives of the Swimmer and the Sailor Flowed Together

SECTION TWO
Reach
Stop Trying to Live, Start Living to Try

Introduction

FRED NELIS

MY JOURNEY—from a heart condition that threatened my life to the transplant that saved it—was preceded by two parental health crises. The first was my mother going to the Cleveland Clinic after giving birth to my youngest sister. At ten, I was just old enough to grasp a hint of understanding of the gravity of my mother's cardiomyopathy, a chronic heart condition caused by her pregnancy. The second occurrence was during my freshman year of college. My dad had a heart attack in the fall. For some reason still unknown, rather than immediately contacting me, Mom sent a letter containing the news.

I was no stranger to heart problems when I began to have them myself. The first indication I had—swim performance issues—was the summer of 1993. I was a competitive swimmer and was asked to join a relay team for a triathlon. My two teammates were accomplished triathletes, their strengths being the bike and run. I was asked to do the swim portion.

In any normal competition, I would have been top five out of the water. Instead, the effort to complete the swim leg was monumental for me. I was hardly able to breathe. The water was very cold, but that couldn't have been the only factor. From that open water swim in June, my stamina seemed to be under attack. As summer turned to fall, my additional efforts during practice failed to produce improvement in performance and depleted my confidence. What was going on?

After repeated trips to the doctor's office, I received two diagnoses: bronchitis, then pneumonia. The direction taken by the medical professionals was to prescribe broad spectrum antibiotics to knock out the infection they thought I had. In reality, however, my breathing problems were the result of fluid pooling in the lungs and around the heart.

Nobody even considered the possibility of heart failure. After all, I had none of the symptoms associated with the disease, such as swelling, shortness of breath, irregular pulse, weight gain, or loss of appetite. However, by this time, I was unable to lie down flat in bed because I could not breathe, and I was sleeping propped up on pillows.

On January 7, 1994, after three sleepless nights, I knew I couldn't continue in this state. It was a Friday, about ten o'clock in the morning, when my wife, Jean, took me to the emergency room at Holland Hospital. I spent the day getting the once-over twice, undergoing endless tests, and answering repeated questions. I twice underwent an echocardiogram that the technician repeated because she couldn't believe the results showed I had heart failure.

It was almost 8:00 p.m. when the cardiologist finally came into the room. I'm still surprised that his report didn't give me a heart attack right then and there. I had idiopathic cardiomyopathy, he said, with an ejection fraction of 10 percent. Normal range for ejection fraction is 55–60 percent. He went on to give me even more cheerful news: I had a 15 percent chance of recovery and would most likely need a heart transplant.

That moment has been forever seared into Jean's and my memories. After the shock of learning, in twenty seconds, that my future was forever changed, it was time to gather up the pieces.

I was 38 years old. And it was the eve of my oldest daughter's tenth birthday.

The full measure of years I'd thought I had ahead of me had suddenly been reduced to a terrifying question mark. I didn't know then

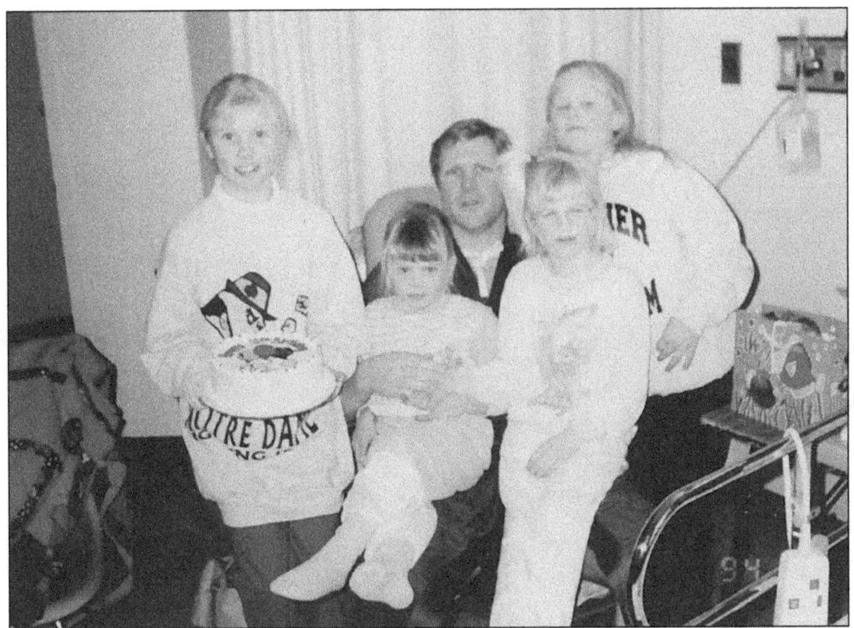

Kelly's 10th birthday celebrated in the hospital, Jan 8, 1994.

that I was about to embark on the toughest—and most interesting—journey of my life.

This is the story of the adventure that lasted just over two decades and ended with the heart transplant that has given me a second chance—in essence, the Jaws of Life rescuing me from the jaws of death. I wouldn't be here today if it weren't for organ donation and Gift of Life, and neither would Gordon Veldman, an old family friend who became a double lung recipient and whose life, in the most fantastic set of circumstances, unexpectedly intersected with mine.

As I write this, Gordon and I have passed our second-year anniversary as transplant recipients. We're not only still here; we're both going strong and are enjoying every minute of our new lives. Unlike cats, we may not have nine of them, but we'll certainly settle for two!

Join us as we relive our remarkable journey of struggle, joy, and always, hope.

Fred Nelis

Introduction

GORDON VELDMAN

"**G**ORDON, wake up and breathe!"

Those were the first words I heard after opening my eyes and looking around the operating room. A major change had occurred in my life in the eleven hours of surgery I'd just undergone. My sixty-six-year-old, hard-as-rubber Alpha-1-damaged lungs had been removed, and a beautiful set of thirty-two-year-old lungs had been installed in their place.

Still groggy from the anesthesia, I put my hand to my chest and found a mass of tubes and gauze. When I closed my eyes, the normal blackness was replaced with boiling waves of tar and flashes of light. Simple thoughts were like billiard balls bouncing around my head. Had I really survived my double lung transplant?

Again I heard the doctor's voice. "Breathe!"

Before the operation, this simple act, one most of us take every second without thinking, was a gargantuan effort. I was operating at less than 15 percent lung capacity, the victim of an inherited degenerative lung disease known as Alpha-1 antitrypsin deficiency. The idea of actually being able to breathe normally again was a dream.

I obeyed the doctor's command. Air filled my new lungs. I took a deeper breath. More air. They were working! I was not only alive—I was reborn.

This book is important because it's a story Fred and I have survived to tell. A wonderful story that highlights what a gift can mean.

Although Fred and I had a relationship before our transplants, coming from the same world and having the same friends, our experience gave us an entirely new relationship. The new heart and new lungs we received define that relationship. We are closer than we could ever have been otherwise—psychologically, physically, and spiritually.

Before our transplants, we were facing imminent death. Today, we are enjoying every minute of new life, a gift so precious that this book is the very best way to express our appreciation.

If there's any message I would like to convey through these pages, it's that your "now" can change in a minute. We don't know what the future holds for any of us. But miracles abound. In my case, I had only mortality to look forward to. Simply trying to breathe was my reality. I was right at the lip of the drain, about to go down, when I got the call that a pair of lungs had become available for me.

To go from gasping for air to raking leaves for two hours this morning is incredible. Thanks to the generosity of my donor, and to the skill and devotion of my remarkable transplant team, I have a "now." The sun on my shoulders, getting a new bike for Christmas, finding my soulmate, the many friends who would come to see me when I couldn't summon the air to say hello, and who are rejoicing with me now…these are just some of the daily blessings for which I never cease to be grateful.

Perhaps the greatest blessing has been love. Where there was once an "I," there is now a "we." I now have someone to live for—my soulmate, Nancy, whom I met after my transplant surgery, and who has transformed my life.

When I see people who complain—and I can be one of those people—I say, to them and to myself, "From now until midnight, enjoy the day."

I hope this book will help you to do that.

And one last thing—I hope this book will inspire you to consider becoming an organ donor. Because you too have the power to give the gift of life.

Gordon Veldman

Preface

TIM HAWKINS

I'LL START WITH A CLICHÉ that I hope will be the last to be found in these pages: The longer I live, the more I grapple and must come to grips with the persistent old adage that, though they may be equally profound, truth is always stranger than fiction.

The story I'm about to tell is beyond my powers of imagination, but living my small portion of it has added a new measure of grace, awareness, and gratitude to my outlook and to my life.

I got to know Fred Nelis and his wife, Jean, and Gordon Veldman and his partner, Nancy Zielinski, in 2015, through my work at Spectrum Health, following the men's successful organ transplants there—Fred for a heart and Gordon for a pair of lungs. Of course, I was initially struck by the incredible coincidence of the reunion of the pair, which this book details. But the irony did not stop there, for, despite some physical and surface similarities, as I got to know them, it soon became apparent that these old family friends were about as unlike in terms of personality, outlook, and temperament as any pair could be.

My first impression was of a gregarious and high-energy Gordon and an ever-smiling Fred, who was perhaps a bit more laid back and reserved. What I didn't fully grasp at the time was Fred's continuing struggle with the moral dilemma of transplant that consumes him to this day and is best summarized in a sign that he hung on the door of hospital room throughout the entirety of his recovery from surgery: "Only the Father knows the balance between grief and gratitude."

However, that understanding would come in time.

AUGUST 1, 2016 was a bright, sunny day in Michigan. The air conditioning happened to be broken in my car, and I drove north on US-131 toward home after work with the windows wide open, the hot air rushing in, and the music blasting on the radio. For that reason, I didn't see or hear my cellphone vibrating until the third or fourth call from my wife. I winced in slight annoyance, realizing I would have to stop for bread or avocadoes before I could get home and enjoy the ritual comfort of sitting under the ceiling fan with a glass of iced tea.

But this call was different. My wife, Ilsy, didn't ask me to stop for groceries. She asked where I was and instructed me to come straight home. She had something to tell me.

She met me in the driveway when I arrived, and I set my briefcase on the hood of the car.

"Just leave it there and come inside," she said.

"Since when do I leave my briefcase outside on the car?" I responded.

"Your sister is dead," were the next words I remember hearing.

I HAD ONLY one sibling, my sister, Kathy. At age 47, while cleaning an upstairs bathroom in the house she had only weeks before moved into and shared with her husband, Josh, and three children Maddie, 17, Sydney, 15, and Charlie, 10, she felt what would have been an excruciating pain in her head and pitched forward onto the linoleum. The pain she felt was her blood transcending the blood-brain barrier following a ruptured aneurysm she knew nothing about. She was dead nearly instantly but would not be found for several hours after failing to pick up Charlie and a friend from golf lessons.

Josh and Maddie received the call from the Kent County Sheriff's Department while beginning the drive home from Ithaca, New York, about 500 miles and more than eight hours away by car. They had been on a college tour. Maddie had been very excited to visit Cornell, though any question of her attending the Ivy League school would be wiped away by the experience of receiving word of her mother's death there.

Josh's brother, Jeremy, tried desperately to book them a flight home from every major city they might pass on their route—Buffalo, Cleveland, Toledo, Detroit. In every case, by the time they would have arrived at the airport and waited for their flight, they would have been home sooner if they had just kept driving. And so they plowed on, mile after excruciating mile, Josh crying in disbelief the entire journey.

I can hardly fathom this journey, though I know it occurred since I spoke to him several times along the way, crying together and encouraging him to keep up his courage and spirits, and reminding him of his important passenger.

The conversation that lingers clear as crystal in my mind, though, pertains to the inquiry he received from Michigan Gift of Life. Kathy was not a registered organ donor. Would he give permission for them to prepare her to become one?

"I don't know what to do, Tim," he choked out. "I don't know what to do. What's the right thing?"

On a day on which there was nothing substantive to be done besides survive, filled with questions that were impossible to answer: How could this happen? Why didn't we know? What could we have done, had we known? How could God be so cruel?

On such a day, this was one small thing I could do, one question to which I could provide a clear and affirmative answer.

"Yes," I answered. "Yes, please give consent. This is the one and only positive thing that can come of this day."

One of my very first texts that afternoon was to Fred Nelis, even before I texted friends and family who had known my sister for years. As he likes to say, I now "had skin in the game" and I wanted him to know what we were doing. I wanted him to know that the reason for the decision was because of him and Gordon. Knowing them had made that much of a difference to me.

I hope that getting to know them and their stories will also make a difference to you.

WHAT FOLLOWS IS a tremendous story of perseverance, faith, joy, and second chances to seize life and live it to the fullest. It is equally the story of the growing awareness of what has been lost and the profound sadness and grief that find the full measure of meaning in providing those second chances.

These themes are human constants and are not necessarily unique to the world of transplant. But suffice it to say that when I first became acquainted with Fred and Gordon, I did not fully appreciate the delicate balance of grief and joy that is unique to this world. Initially, I reveled in the irony and the unexpected twists and turns of a good story, much as I hope the reader shall.

But like my own developing relationship with the men and my own slow dawning of awareness of the full implications of their stories, as you read I hope that you also may find something deeper and more meaningful.

FINALLY, FOR THOSE who would like additional information on the history, myths, controversies, and latest developments in the world of transplant, I direct you to the Appendix, "A Brief History of Organ Transplantation," which can be read prior to, along with, or even after the story of Fred and Gordon's incredible journey. There are many lessons to be taken from this story, but above all, along with Fred and Gordon, I strongly urge you to become an organ donor. There are currently about 114,000 people in the United States waiting for a transplant to save their lives. You can be the person who makes that happen.

Tim Hawkins

THE TRANSPLANT BROTHERS

How the Lives of the Swimmer and Sailor Flowed Together

1

An Amazing Confluence of Events

"The scars from my transplant are an ever-present reminder of the generous gift of a donor and his family, the extraordinary gift of new life."

— FRED NELIS

PERHAPS THE FIRST THING you notice about Fred Nelis (pronounced NEE-LIS) is his smile. Fred is a firm believer in the power a smile holds—to mend a broken heart, melt a frozen heart, or just let a little sunshine in when the rain is getting you down. Fred's smile is big, like he is. He reminds you of an overgrown kid who's really looking forward to something. In Fred's case, that something is life itself.

At age 59, this tall, strapping "Dutch boy," as the Holland, Michigan, native and lifelong resident describes himself, underwent heart transplant surgery. It was not something he ever expected to face; he'd been a competitive swimmer all his life and was in superlative physical condition. That is, until he began having breathing problems in his late thirties. Eventually he ended up in the ER, where tests revealed a sobering diagnosis: idiopathic cardiomyopathy, a progressive heart disease of unknown origin, leading to one inevitable conclusion—advanced, end-stage heart failure. The only remedy was a new heart.

However, because he insisted on maintaining his high level of fitness and continuing to swim, Fred was able to postpone the inevitable for an amazing twenty years. Finally though, his health began to deteriorate, and a transplant could no longer be postponed.

On June 17, 2014, at about 11:00 a.m., Fred was admitted to the Spectrum Health Meijer Heart Center in Grand Rapids. His family and close friends gathered with him. They were tense with anxiety, but he was upbeat as usual, joking away, and soon everyone else was too.

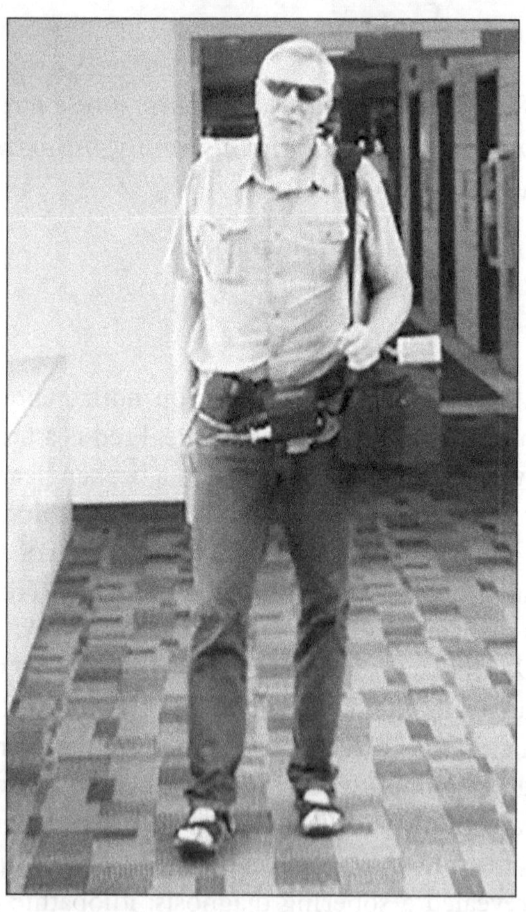

Fred walking into hospital, June 17, 2014

"I remember coming to the hospital at midnight and being in the room as he was getting prepped for surgery," said Fred's eldest daughter, Kelly. "In true Dad fashion, he was joking inappropriately with the nurse and anesthesiologist about getting shaved down. I don't think the nurse knew what to say."

"Dad was very jovial, while the rest of us were like, this is the moment we'd been dreading," said the Nelis' second-eldest daughter, Heather. "He was comedic relief, very lighthearted and joking."

Fred wasn't taken into surgery until nearly 2:00 a.m. When they wheeled him to the OR, the cheerful masks came off, and as his wife, Jean, recalls, "Everyone got emotional." The longest day turned into the longest night for Jean and their daughters—Kelly (30), Heather (28), Lindsey (26), and Jami (25), four beautiful blondes who look like their mom. All had either driven or flown in from around the country.

In the waiting room, they met a woman whose brother was in surgery getting a new pair of transplanted lungs. They had a brief conversation, but the woman wasn't particularly talkative, and soon the Nelis women returned to their own business.

At noon the following day, Fred was transferred to the ICU on the fifth floor of the center. When his family was finally allowed to see him, they weren't prepared for what awaited them.

"He had at least ten infusion pumps and was on a respirator," Jean says. "It was shocking to see him like that."

"He was very pale, lying hooked up to everything," Kelly remembers. "It was hard, seeing him lying there like he was dead, with machines keeping him alive."

Jami, however, wasn't surprised. An OB nurse, her reaction was one of frustration as the day wore on and the breathing tube hadn't been removed. She knew her dad's wish was to have it taken out as soon as possible.

"He was doing well, but by 7:00 in the evening they still hadn't extubated him," she says. "It took longer than it should have. But there wasn't anything I could do, except leave the room before I got really angry at somebody!"

Everyone remembers Fred trying to tell them something. He couldn't talk because of the ventilator, so this became quite the guessing game. They tried getting him to point to letters on an alphabet page, but due to the amount of drugs in his system, his hands were too shaky.

Heather recalls, "Kelly, Lindsey, Jami, and I were all around Dad's bed and he was trying to tell us something. Being the 'kids' and fellow jokesters that we are, we guessed all kinds of things. 'Are you cold/hot?' 'Do you want to get out of here?' 'Are you ready to go for a swim?' Lindsey suggested that he try to write us a message because he was getting frustrated that we didn't understand what he was trying to tell us."

Eventually, after Fred had resorted to charades, Jean put it all together. "You feel like you were run over by a truck?" As Lindsey remembers, "Finally we understood, and Dad sat back with as much of a self-satisfied smirk as he could."

They all burst into laughter.

Then Fred gave the girls sign language for "I love you."

"At that point all jokes were out the window, because we were all in tears," Heather's voice breaks at the recollection.

"We were all crying because he's usually not that demonstrative," Jean says, dabbing tears from her eyes.

At 4:00 p.m., two men came in to administer physical therapy. Fred stunned them all by declaring, "I need to sit up."

"I had to show everyone I was OK. I think I was thinking, I gotta sit up just to show them I'm still alive."

THOSE FIRST HOURS and days of recovery were tough, in particular because, as Fred remembers, "You never knew what was around the corner."

He certainly didn't know what—or who—was literally around the corner—an old friend he hadn't seen in a number of years, Gordon Veldman. It turned out, by sheer coincidence, that Gordon was the double lung transplant recipient whose sister Jean and the girls had talked to in the waiting room. He happened to be recovering in a room just down the hall.

Gordon was a close friend of Jean's brother and sister-in-law, John Vande Bunte and Heide Kenjorski. John and Heide enjoyed hosting gatherings at their cottage on Bills Lake in Newaygo, Michigan. That's where Fred and Gordon first met.

"I first met Gordon when he was doing one of his science presentations at Jean's family cottage on Bills Lake," Fred later recalled. "For a long time, I referred to him as 'Gordon Nye, the Science Guy.'"

They saw each other on those occasions, and over the years had spent numerous summer days and evenings together. But as each grew increasingly ill, it became difficult to get together and they had lost touch. Neither was aware that the other was a transplant candidate.

From her conversation with the woman in the waiting room, Jean knew the man getting new lungs was named Gordon. But she didn't know his last name until her sister-in-law texted her a couple of nights later.

"You'll never guess who called me," Heide said. "Gordon Veldman. He had a double lung transplant at Spectrum. I said, my brother-in-law is there and he just got a heart."

Jean put two and two together. They had been told nothing about Fred's donor, other than he was a thirty-two-year-old man and an athlete. They knew that another recipient was receiving the lungs but had no idea who it was.

What were the odds that two old friends would find themselves in the same hospital, at the same time, across the hall from each other, receiving the organs that would give them new lives from the same donor?

Astronomical would not be an exaggeration. At the very least, it was a definite first for Spectrum Health's Richard DeVos Heart and Lung Transplant Program. As Dr. Michael Dickinson, the program's medical director, admitted, "It's pretty wild. We thought it was quite a remarkable story when it happened."

Gordon Veldman was old by transplant standards—66. But like Fred, he had been in top physical shape as a runner, cyclist, and sailor before he also was struck down by illness. In Gordon's case, by a genetic time bomb—Alpha-1, a degenerative disease of the lungs and liver.

In 1997, at 49, he contracted double pneumonia following a surgery for a knee fracture, and he almost died. Things went downhill from there. A longtime distance runner, he began to notice that his lung capacity seemed to be diminishing.

"I'd do the Lake Stride (a half-marathon following the circumference of Pentwater Lake) and saw that my times were getting slower and slower. I'd always been healthy and never smoked cigarettes. So I didn't know what was going on."

It wasn't until 2007 that doctors were able to pinpoint the cause. Alpha-1 is an inherited disorder, discovered only in the early 1980s and usually found in people of Northern European descent. Like his friend Fred Nelis, Gordon's family came from the Netherlands.

Gordon later discovered that while his two siblings were carriers of the gene mutation that causes the disorder, he was developing the full-blown symptoms of a disease that begins by causing shortness of breath and often leads to damage of the small air sacs of the lungs, and ultimately to lung failure.

This came as a shock, as longevity seemed to be Gordon's most likely genetic condition. His father died at 95, and his mother at 99. But one, or both, of his parents were carriers who had never contracted the disease but who passed it on.

Gordon had always been active. Hiking, running, biking, and sailing were central to his life. That, it turned out, was a good thing when it came to qualifying for transplant surgery.

"Spectrum Health wanted certification for someone they knew would make it through," Gordon said. "Two years ago, at the point where my pulmonologist said that a double lung transplant was possible, things were really bad. I couldn't walk ten feet. My Segway was the only way I could get around town. I couldn't eat a meal because digestion requires oxygen in the blood, and I didn't have the digestive energy. So I had to eat small amounts throughout the day."

Nonetheless, because Gordon had always been so fit, he was able to qualify for surgery. He underwent three months of testing in three weeks. And a month later, he got the call that a pair of lungs had become available.

Gordon's transplant was a success, but not without complications. Since a leading cause of death for new lung recipients is pneumonia provoked by swallowing food into the lungs, he had to learn how to swallow again. In the process, he was allowed no food or water for three weeks and could not leave his bed for the first week. The ordeal was almost unendurable.

"Can you imagine not having a drop of water for three weeks? It was an absolute nightmare. I was so parched my mouth felt like a desert. At one point, I was so desperate I almost called 911 to say, 'These guys are trying to kill me!'"

When Gordon called Heide Kenjorski to tell her about the transplant, he was amazed by her response.

"'I know,' she said. 'I was there.' 'What do you mean?' I said. 'Well, Fred Nelis got a new heart at the same time. His family was in the waiting room with yours.'"

Because Gordon wasn't allowed visitors and couldn't leave his bed, it was a while before the two men connected.

"I saw Fred cruising the hallways with his walker, but I couldn't get his attention," he remembers. "Then I started walking with my Christmas tree of drug paraphernalia and found his room, but the door was always shut. Then John and Heide came to visit me, and I said, 'How is Fred doing?' They said he'd had to have another surgery to remove his LVAD (left ventricular assist device) driveline. So I knew that visiting him wasn't a good idea."

But the two eventually met up and developed a whole new friendship, one that has made them unexpected brothers through a shared donor as well as through a shared mission to tell their story as ambassadors to the general public. Gordon emphasizes the ongoing shortage of suitable organs and seeks to promote the importance of organ donation.

"What we really want to do is to spread the word about organ donation and how important it is to others whose lives depend on it," Gordon emphasizes. "I wouldn't be here now if it wasn't for someone who said yes."

At the end of 2019, nearly 114,000 people in the US were on waiting lists for organ transplants. In the prior year, more than 7,000 people on those lists—about 20 per day—died while awaiting a donated organ to become available for transplant.

While the number of potential recipients on transplant waiting lists has more than doubled over the past twenty-five years, the number of deceased donors has increased by only half. Meanwhile, the numbers of deaths related to the organ shortage has grown in parallel with the waiting list, continuously increasing the gap between supply and demand.

This ongoing situation has led to the development of a number of suggested approaches, ranging from financial compensation for donors to relaxed standards for donated organs to opt-out programs for donors. Science is also producing new approaches to preserving organs for longer periods of time (see Appendix).

Fred emphasizes the moral accountability of the transplant recipient and the duty one has to make the most of someone else's ultimate sacrifice. He brings to mind Tom Hanks's dying Captain Miller in the film *Saving Private Ryan*, who exhorts Matt Damon's Private Ryan to "Earn this!" after losing nearly his entire platoon to bring the soldier home safe to his family. In Fred's case, he is playing both roles simultaneously.

"For a person of conviction, there are moral and ethical questions," Fred says. "Why am I the last one standing? Somebody had to die for me to become a recipient. That is harrowing."

"These questions are not something that transplant recipients take lightly," he adds. "As a recipient, you have a moral and ethical obligation to make the most of your situation. If you don't, it is an injustice to the donor and to the person who is still waiting for an organ. I'm not saying you have to jump the Empire State Building, but you can climb one floor at a time."

"The Transplant Brothers," as they've become known worldwide, are, despite their friendship, a genuinely odd couple. There are a few eerie similarities between them—they're both 6'4", both of Dutch heritage, both remarkably—almost compulsively—active for their ages. But in many ways, their personalities couldn't be more different.

Fred is a longtime businessman, a devout Catholic, a devoted family man with a thirty-seven-year marriage and an incredibly close brood of children and grandchildren. He and his brothers own the Holland-based company Yost Vises, in which he's still active. His kids say that they've never met anyone who works as hard as their father, or who has such a strong faith in God.

Gordon is divorced, with no children, and isn't the least bit interested in organized religion. He retired in 2000 from his job as a Xerox service rep, gave away most of his belongings when he figured he was at death's door, and now lives for the moment. His greatest joy is just getting up and going with his new partner and love of his life. Nancy Zielinski is a retired widow from Chicago, whom Gordon met after his transplant surgery and refers to as "the woman of my dreams."

If Fred is the Establishment, Gordon is the old hippie. Often it seems like they're mystified by each other. But they're closer, through their transplants, than they ever thought they would be.

"There is a very strange bond that's been formed with Gordy," Fred muses. "He's more sentimental than I am. And more eccentric! But we see each other a lot more often now. And we appreciate each other much more, because we know how precious this miracle that we share is."

"Oh, Fred calls me a lot more often now," Gordon smiles happily. "We've developed a unique bond. We give each other our full attention."

And full hugs. Gordon insists that whenever they meet, they hold each other close so that their chests touch, once again uniting their separated organs, at least symbolically.

"Every time I see Fred, we have to go chest to chest," Gordon declares. "Because we are brothers, and that's how brothers treat each other—if they're smart, anyhow."

Fred laughs good-naturedly about the ritual.

"Oh, yeah, Gordy has this hugging thing. I'm not that demonstrative by nature, but I put up with it!"

Nonetheless, when you see photos of the two of them embracing in the "transplant hug," Fred's beaming smile indicates that he just might be enjoying it more than he admits. Gordon's smile also lights up the room.

They definitely have a lot to smile about. Because, not so long ago, they were looking mortality squarely in the eye. Their only hope was that someone would donate the organs they so desperately needed in time to save them.

2

Polar Opposites

If you wanted to pick the perfect dad, a strong presence to provide safety, security, and comfort, you'd pick Fred. But Gordon would be your favorite uncle, the eccentric one who breezes in with all sorts of great adventure stories.

PERHAPS THE MOST INTRIGUING ASPECT of this amazing story of two friends who discovered, purely by chance, that they had received heart and lung transplants on the same day, from the same donor, is the irony that you probably couldn't have found two more different men to join in body and story.

Fred has been involved all his life in the family business, Yost Vises in Holland, Michigan, which he owns with his two brothers. Even today, following his heart transplant, he finds plenty of things to do at the shop. After the nearly forty years his family has owned Yost, the business model has rapidly changed from one of manufacturing to e-commerce, and the Nelises have been forced to adapt. He dreams of someday getting away with Jean for the life of travel and leisure they've put on hold for so many years to build the business and raise a family.

"Don't Fence Me In" could have been written for Gordon. A nomad at heart, he's always on the go and has taken off on many seafaring adventures that are separate books in themselves. He's had his share of both exhilaration and peril, from a year-long sailing voyage to the Bahamas that almost cost him his life, to a 7,000-mile expedition as a crew member on a 1911 tall ship bound for Cape Horn and Antarctica.

Fred lives in a large, lovely house in an upper-crust Holland neighborhood. It's homey and welcoming, with a well-manicured lawn and furnishings that are the essence of good taste.

Gordon's abode looks like something from *The Hobbit*. High on a hill overlooking Pentwater Lake, it's a weathered old cottage with other rough-hewn structures on the premises—a woodworking shop and a shed that houses the wood-burning, smoke-spewing furnace that's the source of heat for the whole property.

Fred's Catholic faith has been a tremendous source of strength for him. Gordon's refusal to embrace organized religion has been his source of strength.

Fred is a conservative, who states his views quietly and politely. Gordon is a liberal, who cheerfully takes any opportunity to verbalize his frustration with the West Michigan Republican establishment—and the establishment in general.

When it comes to their medical conditions, Fred is a model patient, taking his meds according to schedule and generally complying with doctors' orders.

Gordon is more rebellious. He'll square off with the docs over dosages and procedures, and has, as he somewhat ruefully admits, been "taken to the woodshed" more than once, when his defiance has put him in danger of rejection.

Fred isn't into cooking. Gordon is a passionate devotee of home canning and brewing. Friends eagerly look forward to his canned peppers, salsa, dried apples, and Limoncello. During the holiday season, they line up for his prized *banket*, an almond pastry that's a Christmas tradition in the Dutch community.

If you wanted to pick the perfect dad, a strong presence to provide safety, security, and comfort, you'd pick Fred. But Gordon would be your favorite uncle, the eccentric one who breezes in with all sorts of great adventure stories.

In ordinary circumstances, Fred and Gordon wouldn't necessarily have picked each other for best friends. But thanks to their transplant experience, they have become quite fond of each other. They speak often by phone and get together for chat fests at parties, or over a good bottle of wine and Gordon and Nancy's healthy homemade pizza.

In a way they're like conjoined twins, joined at the chest. Literal bosom buddies by chance, not choice, who have learned to appreciate each other's differences as they make the most of every new day they've been given.

FRED IS MAKING vises today.

Yost Vises is a large warehouse with various rooms devoted to manufacturing, storing, and shipping. The industrial environment takes getting used to. The floor is strewn with metal shavings. The huge machines that make the various parts of the vises look like hulking old giants with broad shoulders and great girth, who have been doing their job so long they've become one with it.

"Some of these machines date from the Korean War," Fred observes.

On a gray, snowy day, the shop seems dark, despite the overhead lighting. But Fred is used to the gloomy surroundings. After all, they belong to him and his brothers, who, along with Jean, brother Kevin's wife, Colleen and son, Ryan, are the only employees. This is remarkable, considering the size and scale of their customers. Yost's traditional industrial distribution networks include the federal and state government. More recently, the explosion of e-commerce—including Amazon, Home Depot, and Lowe's—comprises the bulk of their business. The cavernous rooms are filled with parts, finished vises, and thousands of boxes ready for shipping. Yost is a highly successful operation, which has afforded the Nelis family a more than comfortable lifestyle over the years.

Fred has always had a strong sense of duty, to the business and to his family. Even though his heart transplant has given him a daily awareness of the importance of living life to the fullest, he isn't quite ready yet to enter the leisure class. Not that he doesn't enjoy himself. He's grateful for every moment, from being with Jean to playing with his grandchildren to his life's passion, swimming, to, yes, turning out vises. It's all part of the same journey, all the moments woven like varicolored threads into the one beautiful, complex tapestry that makes up a human life.

Fred definitely makes time for fun, but he works it into the larger picture of the business and his dedication to other duties.

GORDON, BY CONTRAST, is formally retired, and like a spirited old racehorse that's gotten a shot of youth hormone, is pawing at the gate. He revels every day in the newfound energy his new lungs have given him. Not a moment goes by, he says, that he doesn't think about where he was prior to his transplant, barely able to move or talk, all his energy devoted to the gargantuan task of taking his next breath.

"To be at the brink of death—to see your dying in your friends' faces—is an unforgettable experience. And to be here today, able to walk, run, bike, able to do the things I never thought I would do again, is a continual miracle."

Gordon is making *banket* today. In the old days, the Dutch pastry—a buttery roll filled with almond paste—was a labor-intensive undertaking involving the rolling out of flaky dough again and again. But Gordon has gotten it down to a science.

"I've been working on the recipe at least ten years," he says. "It's pretty much never fail now. One pound almond paste, 2 cups sugar, 2 eggs. It's the only pastry I make—my ultimate one trick pony."

It's only 11 a.m., but Gordon has already accomplished a full morning's worth of activities. Up at 5 a.m., breakfast, *banket*, and then making library shelves for Patterson Marine in Pentwater. Now he's out on his deck overlooking Pentwater Lake, working on install-ing an old used hot tub that belongs to his partner, Nancy.

"We're going to have a whale of a lot of fun with this," he grins.

Gordon's energy is amazing, not only for a man of 67 but for a man who a year-and-a-half before could barely walk from one end of his living room to the other without stopping for breath. Today, since his double lung transplant, he seems intent on proving there's nothing he can't do.

"Do I have trouble breathing now? Never! Those days are so far gone that sometimes I check myself to make sure. I take a deep breath. That's something I never thought I would ever do again. And it's fantastic. My new lungs are better than anybody's!"

Another thing he never thought he'd live to see was the perfect relationship. Despite his gregarious personality, all his life Gordon had been a loner. Even with two wives and numerous briefer liai-sons, he wasn't, he admits, the relationship type. "I was much too self-centered."

His deteriorating lung disease, however, basically stripped him of his ego. He had to rely more and more on help from others. As he grew closer to death, life acquired new meaning and dimensions. He became more grateful for the smallest things, and more generous. He began giving away all his belongings and saying goodbye to every-thing and everyone. He had probably no more than two months to live when the call came that there were two lungs, just his size, wait-ing for him.

"Knowing that you're going down and there's no bottom," he reflects, shaking his head, "that the only bottom is the end, is stag-gering. There's no off ramp. It changes you forever. There isn't an hour that goes by that I don't think of the terrible inevitability that passed me by. I have to appreciate everything now because I had nothing and suddenly there's a future."

And a future with Nancy. His friends had wanted to introduce him to the slender, attractive widow but were hesitant to do so because he was living on borrowed time. After the transplant, however, the much-anticipated meeting was arranged and it was a classic case of love at first sight.

"I never knew it could be like this," Gordon sighs happily. "Oh, I knew this kind of love existed, but I never dreamed it could happen to me."

Nancy is equally smitten.

"He's my man," she smiles at him adoringly, taking his hand.

They're like teenagers in love. They bike together, hike together, sail together, cook together, and travel the world. At the moment, they're planning a six-week-long jaunt to New Zealand, where they'll rent a camper and drive all over the country. You'd think they were 20.

But for all his youthful enthusiasm, Gordon shows his age in unmistakable, and sometimes sobering, ways. The many post-transplant drugs that are keeping him alive have scary side effects. His skin is brittle and bruises easily. His hands and feet are swollen and numb, the result of drug-related neuropathy. Today, he woke up with an alarming new development—his left eye was swollen and deep red from broken blood vessels. It turns out that his latest rejection medication has increased his ocular pressure to the point of danger.

Fred endures side effects from his meds but doesn't dwell on them. Gordon, by contrast, is on the warpath. He firmly believes that the corporate medical behemoth in America is in bed with the drug companies and ever eager to over-prescribe, over-charge, and basically bleed the public's pocketbooks dry.

"They're profiteers!" he thunders from the bully pulpit of his favorite easy chair. "And I've had it with all the tests, most of which I'm sure I don't need, and the drugs that I don't want to pay for. When I was diagnosed with Alpha-1, my pulmonologist wrote out a prescription for a protein replacement. They get it from plasma. And it was $1000 a month! Once I even paid $10,000 for one infusion. And I never noticed any difference in my condition. But the company kept sending me the stuff. I've got enough boxes to last two lifetimes. To this day I've accused them of operating a total flim-flam."

The more Gordon rants and rails, the more evident it becomes that what he chafes at most about the drugs and tests and constant monitoring is how they've restricted his life. He's itching and aching to run wild, as he did in his twenties and thirties when he sailed the world. But his doctors have him on a short leash and all he wants is to break free.

At the same time, he knows, down deep, that the medical team has his own interests at heart, and that he wouldn't be here today if it weren't for the incredible care and devotion that brought him back to life—and that is still staunchly committed to keeping him going.

"In the end," he sighs, settling down and stretching his long legs, "I'll do what they say. Because I don't have a choice. And because I'll always be grateful to them. In the hospital, whenever anybody came into my room, what they saw was someone who was absolutely appreciative of what they were doing, no matter who they were. Doctors, nurses, food service—it didn't matter. You're alive because of these people. They've given you a future."

3

The Swimmer

"Fred has very high expectations. He is exceptional in how hard he pushes himself. I think he came out of the womb swimming and being an athlete."

—Dr. Michael Dickinson, medical director,
Richard DeVos Heart and Lung Transplant Program

OF ALL THE PEOPLE IN THE WORLD to end up with heart failure, the least likely candidate is probably Fred Nelis.

His fitness level was extraordinary, the result of a lifetime of competitive swimming. In fact, if anything saved his life, before and after his transplant, it was his life in the water.

To Fred, swimming was not just a sport—it was, and is—a passion. But it wasn't his first love. That was football.

Growing up in the 1960s in Holland, Michigan, there weren't a lot of sports to choose from. The big one was Rocket Football, and in their pre-teen years, Fred and his younger brothers were familiar figures on the gridiron.

Unfortunately, in those days before the advent of year-round travel teams, Fred's junior high did not have a football team. In eighth grade, he had to shelve his dreams of football glory and look for another sport to tackle. Unceremoniously cut from the eighth-grade basketball team, Fred was at loose ends, moping around feeling sorry for himself when his parents suggested he try out for the swim team.

"It sure didn't seem so fortuitous at the time," Fred recalls. "But as they say, the Lord works in mysterious ways."

At first it seemed like this was going to be another failure. Fred floundered about, unable to really find his stroke. But the good news for him was that no one was ever cut from the team. By 9th grade, Fred was hooked. Hard work and a breakout season in his sophomore year resulted in a 6th and 11th place finish at the state high school meet, which his high school won.

By his junior year, Fred boasted a 100-yard freestyle time that was a mere half-second off his high school's varsity record. In his senior year, he swam the same freestyle and finished second in the state meet, achieving his school's varsity record in the process. At the same time, he'd gone out for high school football. He played all four years and was all-conference as a senior.

At Kalamazoo College, a liberal arts school of some 1,400 students about an hour from Holland, he went on to realize more football dreams. At 6'4", the strapping young Dutchman made the team and assumed his swimming days were on hold. But crossing campus for classes, he would pass the pool several times a day. And before he knew it, he was back in the water, working out on his own during lunch hour and playing football in the afternoon.

By the end of his college career he had won honors in both sports. He lettered three years in football and was an All-American two-time team captain and four-time all-conference winner in swimming.

Fred set goals for himself that he felt were achievable. The first was to break 50 seconds in the 100-yard freestyle. The second was to earn All-American status for a Division III college. He managed to accomplish both.

Satisfied with attaining his goals, Fred says he never had delusions of grandeur, and did not entertain fantasies of the Olympics, NCAA championships, or world records. The competition in these cases is so intense that the difference between first, second, and third place may only amount to a thousandth of a second.

"These individuals are genetic marvels with a mindset that's as tough as nails," Fred said. "I wasn't in that category, and I didn't want to be. I was comfortable where I was."

As self-deprecating as he may sound, Fred is an intense competitor.

"Fred was very competitive, but it required lots and lots of hard work and lots of early mornings in the pool," recalled Charlotte Nelis, Fred's younger sister and the second child of six. "For someone who doesn't have the natural ability, he put the time into it and had the will to succeed."

Charlotte, who is followed by brothers Kevin, Patrick, and Tom and younger sister Mary, says that Patrick is the best natural athlete in the family. But all of the brothers competed in swimming and pushed each other to be better.

"This is nothing against Pat," said Kevin Nelis. "But Fred always took his sports very seriously."

"Too seriously," chimed in Pat Nelis.

Fred planned to pursue a career in teaching history and coaching swimming, but just two weeks after college graduation in 1977, fate threw him a curve ball. A ruptured appendix landed him in the hospital for three weeks. Interviews for teaching positions were postponed and eventually cancelled because of the abdominal infection that took most of the summer to get over. The robust athlete deteriorated into a weak, scrawny but still towering drink of water who had lost forty pounds of muscle.

However, Fred made the most of his summer in other ways.

Needing a job, he went to work at a local factory making stove piping. The only opening was second shift from 4:30 p.m. to 2 a.m. Fred mentions this as a pivotal time in his life when his spiritual awakening took place.

"Back in the late seventies, TV was off air by about midnight—at least our three channels were silent. What to do at 2 a.m.?" he asked rhetorically.

Fred's solution to insomnia was to undertake a study of the Bible. He spent the remainder of that summer reading the Scriptures faithfully every night, a practice he continues to this day.

"My firm hope and faith are boiled down to the crucifixion scene in St. Luke when the two robbers are crucified next to Christ," Fred said. "At that moment of desperation, when one of them reaches out in faith, Christ tells him, 'Today you will be with me in paradise.' That is the most powerful story in the Bible that really explains the power and the mercy of the Almighty."

Fred's immersion in the stories of the Bible and his exposure to the willfulness and foibles of its characters also led him to another realization: "God must have a sense of humor to continue to deal with this time and time again," he said.

By fall, he was over the worst of his illness and heading back to the pool. Soon he was training hard and looking ahead, not behind. This positive attitude is one of Fred's most valuable assets, because, as he's always maintained, the past remains exactly that: gone and unable to be recaptured or changed. Putting your efforts into the future is a far more efficient use of energy, and to an athlete, it's all about energy.

The ruptured appendix was Fred's first experience with health issues. It would be seventeen years before his next major health crisis: heart failure. Between 1977 and 1994, when he was diagnosed with idiopathic cardiomyopathy, he was swimming an average of 12,000 yards a week, or approximately 350 miles a year.

Swimming had an added bonus for Fred—a wife.

He met Jean Vande Bunte through her brother John. Jean was also a high school and college swimmer, and it didn't take long for her to find lots in common with the handsome champion who was John's cross-town rival in the local meets.

"I knew of Fred Nelis before I ever met him personally," Jean recalls. "He and my brother competed against each other in high school."

Fred and his five younger siblings attended elementary school at Saint Francis de Sales, the local Catholic school in Holland, but went on from there to attend public school at West Ottawa High. Jean's family was literally from the other side of the bridge. They attended Holland High—West Ottawa's biggest rival.

In 1979, the summer after Jean's freshman year of college at Western Michigan University, she held down a job at a local factory in Holland. She also worked out with a group of local college-age swimmers at Hope College's pool. Fred's younger brother, Pat, was also a part of that swimming group.

"I knew Pat from past AAU (now USA Swimming) swim meets," Jean recalled. "Fred was going to be the volunteer coach for our practices, which were held in the late afternoon after everyone was done working.

"Pat introduced us and a few weeks later we went out on a double date with him and his girlfriend," Jean said. "A few days later, Fred asked me out, and by the end of the summer we were practically inseparable."

What attracted her to her future husband?

"Fred was just so funny," Jean said. "He had this wonderful sense of humor."

Fortunately, Fred got serious long enough to propose to his beautiful blonde just four months after they met. They married in 1981, and by 1989 were the happy parents of four beautiful blonde girls. But even with a full family schedule and work at Yost Vises with his brothers, Fred still made time to swim.

It could well have been the smartest thing he ever did. Later, his ability to commit to a consistent training regimen and his insistence on continuing to swim in the face of a deteriorating heart condition probably made the difference between being a fair prospect and an excellent transplant candidate.

That extraordinary degree of self-discipline was a quality instilled in him by his parents, who were the embodiment of no-nonsense fortitude.

Fred was born on January 19, 1955. His mother, Kathryn (Kay) (nee Murphy), a woman of strong Irish-Catholic heritage, left her career as an RN to become a stay-at-home mom. His father, Fred Sr., owned and operated, with his father Harry and brother Harry, two legendary Holland institutions: Nelis' Dutch Village and Nelis' Tulip Farm. Located on a 40-acre site at the corner of US-31 and James Street, Dutch Village began in the 1950s as a retail outlet for bulbs and souvenirs and grew into a small, Dutch-themed amusement park. Over the years it added a replica Dutch village and attractions including costumed klompen dancers, street organs, a carousel, carillon bells, and heirloom quality gifts and souvenirs.

Kay was from the farm country of Mount Morris, near Flint, on the eastern side of the state. A pretty, petite ball of fire who ran the household with a loving but stern hand, Kay insisted that her children attend Mass every Sunday, no excuses accepted. This is a tradition that Fred does his best to maintain, regardless of whether he is traveling or even when riding his four-wheel ATVs in the boondocks of Northern Michigan.

"Mother was a woman of relentless faith in God," Fred said. "I cannot recall *ever* missing Sunday Mass."

Fred's father, Fred Sr., was taciturn, proud, tough, and hardnosed, yet completely devoted to his family. Despite being a man of few words, when he spoke he was widely respected. His counsel was valued by his family, peers, and even church leaders—and his generosity was legendary. He was also one of those gritty old-school men of his generation who ignored sickness and pooh-poohed pain—perhaps to his grudging regret.

"We could talk with him, but his analogy was, 'You can do what you want, but if you put your hand on the burner you will know that it's hot,'" said Kevin Nelis.

Yet there was also a softer side to Fred Sr.

"While Mom was powerful in faith, Dad was exceedingly generous," Fred said. "One story I recall concerned the time that our grade school couldn't make its monthly payroll. Dad stepped forward and took care of it."

In 1994, when Fred Jr. received the devastating diagnosis of idiopathic cardiomyopathy, he was just 38 years old. His parents' concern, care, and support were critical to his emotional health, and his ability to remain both strong and optimistic.

At the time of Fred's diagnosis, his parents had recently purchased an Airstream travel trailer. Fred Sr. had sold his share of the Dutch Village to his brother Harry in the mid-1970s, started another business, Yost Vises, and was ready to hand over the reins to the next generation and retire. Fred Sr. and Kay were excited about traveling, spending time together, and leaving the grueling Michigan winters for the warmer climate that was much kinder to Kay's severe rheumatoid arthritis. But when Fred was diagnosed, she insisted on putting off their departure until his health stabilized. Nobody at the time realized just how precious those years would be for them.

Fred Sr. had suffered most of his life from familial high cholesterol. He had his first heart attack in 1973, underwent the first generation of stent procedures in the early 1990s, and finally had bypass surgery in 1995.

In 1998, Kay was diagnosed with lung cancer. True to character, she fought her prognosis with courage and faith. Like her husband and now her oldest son, she had, after all, spent most of her adult life battling devastating illness without complaint.

In 1964, at age 32, following the birth of her youngest child, Mary, Kay suffered heart failure, a result of pregnancy-induced cardiomyopathy. The condition nearly killed her, and she lived with it for the rest of her life. While the new baby spent the first six months of her life being cared for by her uncle James Murphy and his wife, Avis, Kay fought for her life at Cleveland Clinic with one thought in mind:

"I've got to live long enough to deal with my family, take care of family, raise my family," Charlotte said. "She wasn't about to let anybody else do that. And she would never draw attention to her condition, would never want to be known as an invalid."

This persistence and acceptance in the face of adversity is a trait that she and Fred Sr. succeeded in passing down to their children.

"You are given your plate and deal with it and do the best you can," said Charlotte Nelis. "It's not about 'poor me' or 'oh woe is me.' Our parents modeled it. Okay, you have a twist in the road here. What do you do? How do you work with that?"

"We use the terminology that Fred is a workhorse, a plow horse," said Pat Nelis. "He puts his blinders on and he stays focused and keeps working. He's been a plow horse for 55 years."

This characteristic is noticeable to outsiders and to friends like Jill Caesar, a long-term neighbor to Fred and Jean, who is more like family.

"If you knew Jean and Fred, you'd never know they'd been through all of this," said Caesar, referring not only to Fred's cardiomyopathy, but also to Jean losing her mother to brain cancer at a young age and her own serious bout with colon cancer. "They don't get discouraged. They don't deny what is happening, but they just have such positive outlooks and they don't give in to despair."

Both Caesar and Charlotte Nelis chalk up much of this stoicism and fortitude to the couple's strong foundation of faith.

"Faith has played a strong role in our family," said Charlotte Nelis. "We all practice yet. It comes down to: This is what we've got. This is what God gave to us. How are we going to deal with it? How are we going to make it better?'"

Kay's faith, however, would be severely tested—in a way that took Fred Jr. by complete surprise.

Following her cancer diagnosis, in true Kay fashion, she was determined to do everything medically possible to attack this foul intruder in her life. The next two years included partial lung removal, chemo, and radiation therapy.

Not once, said Fred, did he recall her losing her resolve to beat her cancer. However, one quiet morning he stopped in to chat with his mom, and to his amazement, she began the conversation by announcing how furious she was with God.

"But it wasn't about her situation; it was about mine," Fred recalled. "Shocked, I listened as she let loose with both barrels. How could a loving God drop such a heavy burden on me? My four beautiful daughters might be without a father. Jean would be left alone."

In essence, she was giving God a scolding. "OK, Lord, I can handle what you've dished out to me. But why give my son a big helping too? Shame on you!"

But she also had something else to announce. At this juncture in her cancer, which had spread, she had two options: to continue with the chemo that had so weakened and ravaged her, or simply stop treatment in favor of whatever quality of life she could maintain until the end. She had decided, she told Fred, to continue the treatments for his dad, so that they could have a few more months together.

"To go through all that suffering and emotional turmoil just for the hope of a few good days among the bad weeks demonstrated a love inadequately explained by the best minds and authors of history," said Fred.

Kay's fight finally ended in 2000, when she put an end to her treatments and prepared for the inevitable. In accordance with her wishes, she spent her final days at home, where all of her children took turns waiting vigil at her bedside. The most heartbreaking moment came in the midst of a morphine haze, when she opened her eyes and looked at her husband, who had been unswerving in his attention and care.

"Don't take too long," she whispered to him. "I'll be waiting."

She passed away quietly not long afterward.

After his mother's death, Fred watched his father deteriorate. Kay didn't have long to wait. Fred Sr. joined her the following year, after suffering a heart attack while golfing with his best friend.

Living through the deaths of both his parents in such a short space of time was a monumental experience for Fred, in more ways than one. There was, of course, the terrible grief at the loss of such an integral support system in his life. But there were also several vital lessons he learned, about the tremendous power of true love, true faith, and the commitment to fight for life.

These lessons would steady and guide him when it came time for him to confront his own mortality. Above all, they were reminders that his parents were still and would always be there, through the wisdom they passed on to him.

"Powerful in prayer, faith, and generosity our parents showed us how to live and more importantly how to die," Fred reflected. "They gave me their name, their love, and their God. What more could I have asked for?"

He may not have asked for it, but Kay's living embodiment of commitment, fortitude, and determination found its way into the next generation of Nelises and into her grandchildren as well.

Dr. Michael Dickinson, Fred's cardiologist and medical director of the Richard DeVos Heart and Lung Transplant Program, said Fred's attitude, athleticism, and determination have contributed to his positive outcome.

"I think he came out of the womb swimming and being an athlete," Dr. Dickinson told *Spectrum Health Beat*. "Fred has very high expectations. He is exceptional in how hard he pushes himself. This helped his outcome. To perform at a high level athletically, it takes somebody motivated who is willing to work at it."

Krista Veine works as a transplant manager at Spectrum Health's Richard DeVos Heart and Lung Transplant Program, and has known Fred since 2013.

"It is interesting, as a manager, I don't often meet every patient. I typically get to meet patients with issues or problems or ones who are friendly or ones who are bigger than life," she said. "Fred was a bigger than life character; he has a big personality and is very driven and very motivated.

"In fact," she added, "he was one of the most motivated patients we have ever had, as far as knowing his goals and setting out to achieve them, and you'd better be along for the ride."

Looking back on all that Fred has experienced, the high expectations and intense motivation turned out to be essential attributes enabling him to survive and thrive in his twenty-year journey from cardiomyopathy diagnosis, to LVAD (left ventricular assist device), to transplant and recovery.

4

The Sailor

"When the motor shuts off, the quiet takes over. You, the lake, and the boat are one, all is well, and you're sailing to yet another adventure… Water is the last endeavor of pure nature in this world."

— GORDON VELDMAN

IF FRED WAS A BORN SWIMMER, Gordon was a born sailor. The waves held him in their spell. In fact, he had something of a mystical relationship with the water, an inexplicable fascination that began as far back as he can remember.

"When I was growing up in Grand Rapids, our family had no boat and no marine connection," Gordon said. "But I'd draw boats and dream about them. I felt like a sailor from the beginning; it's something I can't explain."

And something he couldn't explain to his family, a stern bastion of the Christian Reformed Church, which along with the Reformed Church in America is one of two North American branches of the former Dutch Reformed Church, a religion that, at least in the 1950s, didn't indulge dreams or flights of fancy.

"I grew up Dutch Reformed, where love is not so much emotion as a triad. If I love my sister, I'd say, 'I love you because I love Jesus and Jesus loves you; he's the linchpin of love,'" Gordon explained. "So you don't really love the person—you love them through Jesus. So it abdicates responsibility for emotional love.

"As a result, I never felt the warmth of parental love," he added. "Oh, my parents were good people. But they never really showed love. They were simply fulfilling their duty of raising a Christian family."

Gordon was born November 28, 1947, in Grand Rapids, to Raymond and Grace (Bolthouse) Veldman. Raymond was an early employee of renowned, self-taught engineer, inventor, and business-man Bill Lear, best known for the invention of the Lear Jet and the 8-track audio tape cartridge.

Gordon's father worked as an equipment repairman in one of Lear's test laboratories, though Gordon never talked with him much about it. Despite both parents' longevity, each living well into their nineties, Gordon says that he never really knew them very well.

"My father was dominated by my mother, so I really don't know who he was. He was monochromatic—no fishing trips or anything," Gordon recalled years later. "My mother was really dominant but not very expansive—oars always in the water and always pulling forward."

The Dutch Reformed Church was forged in the fires of Calvinism, as John Calvin's writings and teaching came to be known. The French, sixteenth-century Reformation theologian helped establish and lead a theocracy in Geneva. In his writing, he proposes a system of theology that attempts to explain the relationship between God's sovereignty and man's responsibility in the matter of salvation from death and eternal damnation.

Unfortunately for Gordon, he was not taught or did not absorb the larger context of Calvin's teachings, but instead focused on the tenets of the total depravity of man and the idea of limited atone-ment, which holds that Jesus died only for the "elect," or for those who were "predestined" to be saved in the beginning of time.

About the doctrine of predestination, Calvin wrote in his *Commentaries on Election and Predestination*: "It seems harsh to many to think that God chooses some and rejects others, and does not consider men's worth, that by his own free will he chooses whom he pleases and moreover rejects others. But what is this scruple except a desire to call God to order and subject him to their judgment?"

For Gordon, the emotional coldness of teachings that reduced Calvin to predestination and depravity was soul numbing. Coupled with undiagnosed dyslexia, it affected his ability to learn and to connect with others.

He was expelled from his Christian elementary school in third grade for non-attention and disciplinary issues and was briefly sent to public school, which, he said, was the best thing that ever happened to him.

"In public school, I was immediately put in speech therapy, and I loved my teachers," Gordon recalled. "I don't remember any of my Christian teachers, but I remember vividly my public school teachers."

In the long run, however, Gordon simply wasn't suited to the world of academia. His gifts were nurtured outside of the traditional educational milieu. He had a talent for woodworking, building, and discovering the natural world through experimentation that he would later take into schools, introducing kids to the magical world of science through games and devices that ignited imaginations and delighted young minds.

Later in life, he would develop myriad interests that included kayaking, biking, running, woodworking, mechanical tinkering and inventing, cooking and canning, travel, and above all, time spent with friends, for Gordon is the ultimate extrovert.

"He delighted in unique stuff," said longtime friend, Chrissie Hall. "Gordon always said that his parents made him feel like a loser, and I think he had a desire to learn about things to prove them wrong."

"He is brilliant, and can figure out how things work, but he is extremely dyslexic," said former wife Beverly Fogarty. "For that reason he doesn't like to write letters and emails. He has a very good memory too, and can remember facts, especially anything scientific."

"Gordon is always trying to invent or fix something, and he is often wrong, but always sure of himself," said longtime friend Heide Kenjorski. "You know he is a little crazy, but he is so smart that even if you don't always believe him, you want to."

Despite his desire to share his experiences with friends, his interests, talents, and iconoclastic views are totally his own and form the essence of what some friends refer to as "Gordwardian Theories" or "The Gordwardian Way." This was evident even at a young age.

"Gordon was a square peg in a round hole and never quite fit in growing up," said his sister Margo, who is five years Gordon's junior. "He was super bright in the science world and the mechanical world, but had more difficulty with other things.

"Maybe he got some of that from Dad," she said. "Dad came from the age where they fixed everything instead of replacing it.

"I don't think my parents ever understood him," she added. "But he always told them he loved and cared for them and they told him that they loved him as well."

Gordon and his older brother, Tom, shared a bedroom in the basement, and according to Margo, since they were so unlike each other, the two brothers had a lot of disagreements.

"Tom was always into sports and school and girlfriends," she said. "Things came easier for him. Gord was always into science. He made smoke bombs in the basement while his books would sit open unread."

Gordon finished high school a year late, graduating with the East Christian High School class of 1966. By 1968, he was still living in Grand Rapids and trying to sort out his future. That year was a pivotal one in terms of US involvement in the war in Vietnam with the Tet Offensive, the countercultural protest movements sweeping the nation, and the presidential race that would impact US involvement in Southeast Asia for nearly another decade. Lacking a student deferment, Gordon was drafted into the US Army.

Looking back on his life, Gordon admits that he has had both extremely good and extremely bad luck. If losing the genetic lottery with his Alpha-1 diagnosis is a prime example of the latter, his experience in the Army is that of the former.

While thousands of boys of his generation were drafted that year to fight and die in the rice paddies and rain forests of Southeast Asia, Gordon's military experience was a life-affirming turning point in his life. It was also an ironic one, as the defiant young recruit with an aversion to authority and the establishment eventually came to credit the US military, and one individual in particular, for the discovery of his true inner self.

Gordon describes himself at the time he entered the military as an "unmotivated, physical marshmallow with no self-pride." Twenty-four months later, after being stationed in West Germany and driving an oil tanker throughout Europe, he emerged as a Spec/4 with pride, a high degree of physical fitness, and, perhaps for the first time in his life, a belief that he might amount to something.

"The most influential person in my life was a young, black drill sergeant, Sgt. Williams," Gordon recalled. "He saw my potential and got me through basic training. Without his tutelage, I would probably have been a suicide."

Sgt. Williams would stand behind Gordon during basic training and literally whisper into his ear, "Veldman, how are we going to get you through this?"

"What an amazing thing he did for me, realizing that the standard tactic, yelling, was not going to help," Gordon said. "Those six weeks of basic training did more for my character development than sixteen years of Christian education.

"What does it take to make an empathetic person? It takes someone with empathy to pass it on," Gordon said. "Williams could tell that I was so damn fragile I couldn't handle the brutality so much loved by the military."

As a result of his experience, Gordon started reading more broadly and got hooked on the excitement of travel, taking advantage of being stationed in Germany to trek throughout Europe, ski in the Alps, and have the time of his life.

"I realized I wasn't as bad as I thought," Gordon said. "This marshmallow Christian kid became a person who could say, 'Yes, I can do that,' thanks to the US Army."

After his service ended, he was somewhat at loose ends, flipping burgers at a fast-food restaurant back in Grand Rapids when he landed an opportunity that would provide employment for the rest of his working life.

Gordon answered a recruiting ad to test and interview to become a service repair representative for Xerox. He knew that he would have no trouble passing a hands-on examination but was equally aware from his academic career that a written test would likely prove problematic. The affable Gordon quickly established a rapport with the recruiter, who, in another stroke of good fortune, allowed the dyslexic applicant extra time on his written test. Granted this accommodation, he wound up acing the test and was hired as a Xerox repair representative.

He had found his niche.

According to his second wife, Beverly, Gordon had one of the lowest parts budgets of any repair rep in the country because he could fix the copier components himself instead of ordering new parts. He also had an engaging, outgoing, likeable personality that brought him recognition and appreciation from clients. In the Holland area, he became known as "Xerox Man." He won awards, was feted by the company, and was flown around the country to conventions and events to celebrate his success.

He also finally had the income he needed to pursue the dream he'd never abandoned: to become a sailor. He ordered a 16-foot kit boat and assembled the craft. Over the next decade he acquired bigger boats, and in 1979, he bought his Islander 26, a 26-foot sloop that he christened *Just Dandy*, because when he was checking it out for the first time, a man came along and observed, "Isn't that just dandy!"

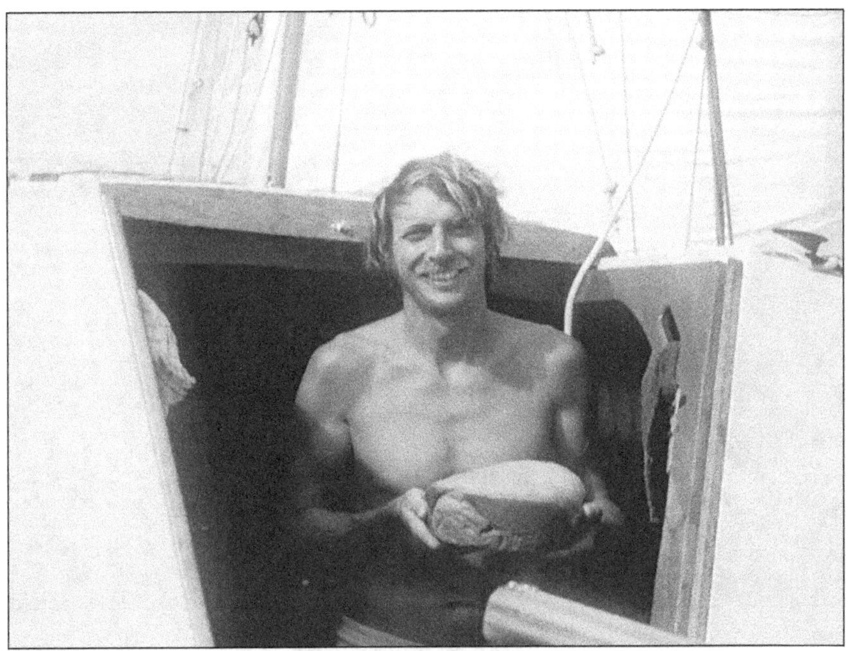

Gordon on *Just Dandy*

The following year, Gordon and his first wife, Carol, whom he had married in 1970, embarked upon the adventure of a lifetime: a year-long cruise to the Bahamas.

A two-week Bahamas sailing trip with friends in the late 1970s sparked the couple's passion. They decided they wanted more time there and spent three years preparing for the journey. The voyage would take them from Lake Michigan down the Illinois River to the Mississippi River, the Gulf Coast, Florida, and finally, their destination. Much of the journey between the Mississippi and the Caribbean would take place through the Intracoastal Waterway, a 3,000-mile inland waterway along the Atlantic and Gulf coasts, consisting of natural inlets, saltwater rivers, bays, and artificial canals. Upon leaving the Waterway, along the Florida Gulf Coast, and after setting sail from Miami, the couple would face the potential hazards of travel on the open sea.

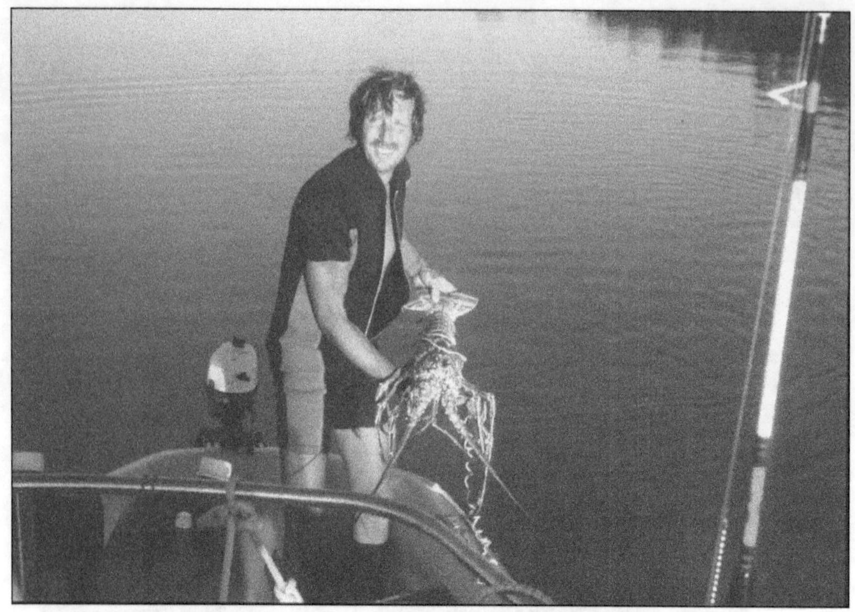

Gordon catching lobster

After much wangling, Gordon was able to obtain a leave of absence from Xerox, and Carol quit her secretarial job at Grand Valley State University in Grand Rapids.

An old scrapbook, yellowed with age, chronicles their experience. The cover page proclaims: "Now Showing: Bahamas Voyage. Slide Show of the Ten Month Voyage from Holland, Michigan, to the Bahamas on a Small Sailboat. Narrated by Author/Adventurer Gordon Veldman." At the bottom of the page is a photo of the beaming couple—he, with tousled brown hair and a moustache, looking even younger than his 32 years; she, blond, petite, and extremely pretty, both of them laughing with carefree abandon.

"About five years ago my wife and I decided that we were the typical American couple," Gordon told a reporter from the *Milwaukee Journal*. "Seeing each other for twenty minutes a day and talking to each other about ten minutes. That is when we made a commitment to start doing things we like to do.

"I work to live, not live to work," he said.

Although acquaintances expressed skepticism about the voyage and its impact on their careers, Carol told the *Holland Sentinel* in a pre-trip profile, "Our friends believed us because most of them are our sailing buddies."

To gain their sea legs and get accustomed to full-time life on the water, Gordon and Carol planned to spend a week or two visiting destinations along the Lake Michigan coast. The first page of their sailing log is dated September 15, 1980. The couple set sail "downwind" from Holland at noon and docked in Grand Haven at 6:30 p.m., spending "$6.25 for dockage, $7.25 for dinner, $1.20 for ice, and $4.00 for 'goodies.'" The weather was described as "Light airs, partly cloudy. Cool."

Despite this innocuous start to their voyage, the ensuing scrapbook pages tell a story neither of them could ever have imagined.

Gordon had made it through two years of military service unscathed, but seven days into their voyage he suffered a grievous wound that would set the couple's plans back by several months. After sailing across Lake Michigan, resting below deck, tied to the sea wall of the Milwaukee Yacht Club on September 22, Gordon was shot on his boat by a young, off-duty Marine.

"Sailing Adventure Halted by Another Adventure," read the headline in the *Holland Sentinel*. "Barely on the first leg of their year-long sailing adventure to the Bahamas, Gordon and Carol Veldman of Holland have met up with some serious obstacles.

"'Our boat has bullet holes the size of a half-dollar, and I've been shot in the rear by a Marine,' is how Gordon, 32, summed up the situation. A 19-year-old Marine was charged with negligent use of a weapon and criminal damage to property Monday morning for allegedly wounding Veldman while firing a 30.06-caliber high-powered rifle into the couple's moored sailboat while they were resting below deck."

Gordon was rushed to Milwaukee County General Hospital and listed in satisfactory condition. The bullet had torn through the muscles in his buttocks and wounded him in the upper leg and side of his torso.

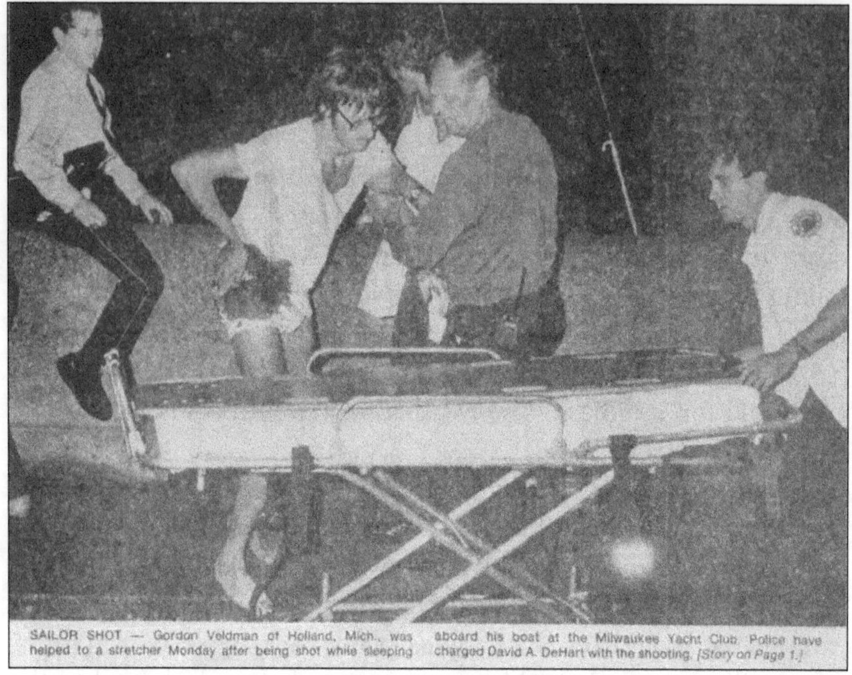

SAILOR SHOT — Gordon Veldman of Holland, Mich., was helped to a stretcher Monday after being shot while sleeping aboard his boat at the Milwaukee Yacht Club. Police have charged David A. DeHart with the shooting. [Story on Page 1.]

Gordon shot

The story made fourteen Midwest newspapers and the network news. Coverage of the event describes the young Marine, David de Hart, at home on leave from his base in Yorktown, Virginia, and drunkenly engaged in "target practice" with friends.

Gordon told the *Grand Rapids Press* afterward that Carol heard two shots aimed in another direction, and, "Then she heard someone say, 'Let's shoot at this boat.'" Carol's screaming woke him up, and in the darkness of the boat the pair could see a new stream of light each time one of thirteen bullets pierced the fiberglass hull.

One of the bullets that found its way into Gordon's leg also hit a feather pillow so that the cabin of the boat was a gory scene of blood and feathers, almost appearing as if a tar and feathering had taken place.

Gordon knew the ambulance gurney would not fit into the boat's cabin, so he decided to walk out into the glare of the TV cameras and photographers' lights, which can clearly be seen in coverage of the event.

"That was my fifteen minutes of fame," said Gordon. "I still have a huge flesh wound. To be shot on your boat seven days out on a year adventure by a U.S. Marine is quite an achievement!"

It was his first brush with mortality. But he was young—and he was Gordon, ever indefatigable, fueled by an unquenchable wanderlust that would become the driving force of his life.

5

The Sailor: Uncharted Waters

"We built a nice fire on the high hill and first fried the fritters and then had the fish, cornbread, salad, and spuds…We had a great time and everyone was stuffed… We swapped a lot of great stories and some songs. It was a super nice night and we could see lightning way off to the east."

—Gordon Veldman

ON THE CUSP of his and Carol's Bahamas trip in October 1980, Gordon was recovering from a huge gunshot wound, the scars of which he would bear (and proudly bare to his closest friends) for the remainder of his days. A traumatic event that might sink the plans of most adventurers barely put a dent in Gordon's enthusiasm.

"Sailor Won't Let Bullet Scuttle Plans for Trip," reported the *Milwaukee Journal.* "'Too much effort and thought has been put into this trip to toss it aside just because of one quirk,' says Gordon Veldman."

Both Gordon and the boat required some emergency repairs before setting sail again. Lifelong sailing friend Steve Wolff of Holland went to Milwaukee, performed some emergency repair work, and sailed

Just Dandy back to Holland where it underwent $1,500 in repairs at Bay Haven Marina. There were thirteen holes in the hull, though luckily none below the water line. The high-powered rifle had caused extensive damage to the interior of the boat, however.

Gordon underwent a skin graft on October 3 at St. Mary's Hospital in Grand Rapids to close his large wounds. The "Bahamas Voyage" scrapbook is filled with newspaper clippings, get-well cards, Gordon's hospital wrist band, repair receipts, hospital discharge papers, and insurance claim forms. But it is two spiral notebooks that served as the *Just Dandy*'s sailing logs that best tell the rest of the story of what happened over the next ten months.

Gordon and Carol set sail again on Tuesday, October 21, accompanied for the first leg of the journey by Steve Wolff. They made Chicago the next morning, but with little wind had motored as much as sailed, and running low on gas, required a tow through the first lock into the Chicago River and the city.

Gordon's all-caps printed (and "creatively" spelled) log entries (edited for clarity) show his reaction to the sudden change of sailing from the open water of Lake Michigan to sailing through downtown Chicago.

"What a trip to go through the center of a city as big as Chicago," he writes. However, after lunching at a downtown bar called The Greenery, he adds, "We all were glad we were not like the people in that bar."

Typically, it is Gordon who notes the parties and good times the three young sailors were invited to along the way. With his infectious personality, the youthful, attractive trio had no trouble meeting other sailors and yacht club members who wanted to hear about their adventures and plans for the Bahamas.

But it is Carol's neat cursive handwriting that inscribes most of the early log entries, and she includes a multitude of details from this first part of the trip. She mentions the small towns along the Illinois River, such as Hennepin and Seneca with "three bars, a grocery store and a bank," the limestone cliffs of Pere Marquette State Park, an archaeological site near Kampsville with more than a million "Indian relics," and a beautiful lodge built in the 1930s with two fireplaces where "Gordy had catfish."

The giddiness of being out on the open water, free from the responsibilities of the workaday world, is palpable in her observations of the autumn leaves and the places where they docked to have an ice cream and mail postcards back home.

The only damper thus far had been the weather, which was cold and rainy that first week. But that was sure to change soon. By October 29, they had reached Grafton, Illinois, where the Illinois River flows into the Mississippi. "From here on it's South all the way," reads that day's entry.

On the 30th, having cleared one final lock and entered the mighty waterway, they anchored in sight of the Gateway Arch in St. Louis.

In St. Louis, Gordon and Carol said goodbye to Steve Wolff. After shopping, eating a Chinese dinner, and having drinks at Trader Vic's, they left him in the care of a "lady friend." "He is a good friend and a rare person," Gordon writes in one of his last log posts for a while.

Wolff was a kindred spirit and Gordon would cherish that friendship for many years. Even after becoming separated by geography later, Gordon would make the ninety-minute drive to Holland from his new home up the Lake Michigan coast in Pentwater to join Wolff's regular Thursday night sail as often as he could.

MEANWHILE, THE MISSISSIPPI presented a host of new challenges for Gordon and Carol as they made their way alone toward New Orleans and the Gulf of Mexico. The river was low that time of year and night-time anchorages were hard to find. Many tributaries where they might find shelter for the night were dried up or too low to enter safely. Often they took to anchoring behind "wing dams," man-made rockpiles deflecting the current to the main navigation channel.

On Halloween night, they found shelter in the Kaskaskia River, where they listened all night to the Army Corps of Engineers dredging the river. The log book describes a night of "clanging, banging and racket" throughout which the dredge boat would blow off steam as rocks and other debris clattered through the pipes of the dredging equipment. It was a very noisy place to anchor, but at least the river was calm. They emerged the next day to find the deck covered with flying spiders and cobwebs.

After anchoring for the night of November 10 in a small river cut north of Greenville, Mississippi, *Just Dandy*'s trip line was swept under the boat by the current and wrapped around the propeller as they hoisted anchor the next morning. Gordon had to tie himself to the boat and dive down into the strong current to free the propeller.

Despite these mishaps, the couple seemed happy. Gordon, ever the capable handyman, was able to diagnose and repair any malfunction thus far, the weather had turned warm and Carol writes that both were quite sunburned ("How strange in November"). As they motored and sailed south over the next couple of weeks, they frequently ran into fellow sojourners they had met upriver.

Carol writes that Thanksgiving 1980 in New Orleans was "a beautiful day." Yet starting with the entry on December 4, we rarely hear again from Carol, our main narrator to this point. Gordon's all-caps gives way to his more gnomic, inscrutable handwriting, which takes over from Carol and continues to the end of the first notebook and completely fills the second notebook. Gordon paints a picture at times ecstatic and celebratory and at times bleak and hopeless. In addition to the sunny times ahead, there would be days and nights filled with danger, conflict, and turmoil.

The next week through the Intracoastal Waterway was sunny and uneventful, with Gordon trying his hand at shrimping near Dauphin Island. But a new challenge awaited the couple as they reached the Florida Panhandle port of Apalichicola, where they would set out on a direct diagonal route for St. Petersburg, across the open water of the Gulf of Mexico.

On December 11, they observed and noted a pod of porpoises playfully swimming before embarking on their crossing that evening. The porpoises' behavior contrasted sharply with the mood of the couple. As night fell, the wind began picking up from the north, both were apprehensive, and Carol was stricken with seasickness.

"Darkness fell and Carol's apprehension increased 10-fold," Gordon writes. "During the night, the sky lit up like daylight and a large meteor flashed overhead."

At one point during the night crossing, Gordon became lost and disoriented.

"Carol is very disenchanted and we are having a bad time of it," he wrote. "I am suffering from lack of sleep and am very strung out.

"Things hit their lowest point at that time. Carol was despondent and crying and I was not much better," he says, later. "At that point I realized our trip was in grave danger and I wanted to quit!"

Nonetheless, they survived the crossing, returning to the relative safety of the Intracoastal to cross the Florida peninsula near Fort Myers, where the couple began "seeing more and more boats as we get into the thick of boating world." Gordon was ecstatic to meet another sailor who also had the distinction of being shot on his own boat. "Just one of the great people you meet along the way," he writes.

As they reached North Palm Beach on December 23, Gordon celebrated: "For the first time this trip we swam in the Atlantic Ocean. Super!"

The next day, however, the boat stalled and Gordon spent most of the day fixing it and fighting with Carol.

"I sure wish we could understand each other better," he writes. "I think we have bigger problems than we both will admit…I would like to go on alone but I don't think that is possible."

On the 25th, they got up and wished each other Merry Christmas. Neither had gotten the other a gift. They each called their parents.

"I think Carol feels very bad today that she is not home with family," he writes. "That is one of the worst things about this sailing game. But you can't take everyone with you."

Despite the melancholy Yuletide, there were sunny, carefree days ahead, evoking the fantasies of would-be castaways and adventurers in offices, factories and classrooms around the world. They were also joined for several weeks on December 29, by Michigan friends Bob and Linda Sperling, which added some variety to the close quarters.

On January 2, 1981, accompanied by the Sperlings, the couple set sail from Miami, across open water, bound for Bimini. Gordon's giddiness at reaching the islands is palpable in his entries. *Just Dandy* appears to be "the first of the river group" to reach Bimini, the fishing was good, and they celebrated their successful crossing by having drinks at a bar Hemingway frequented in the 1930s.

Much of the rest of the sailing journal is dedicated to the mundane, day-to-day preoccupations of living at sea: locating the best anchorages; keeping track of expenses; noting the best places to find replacement parts or to buy ice, fresh water, and gasoline; celebrating a store with fresh eggs and low prices or a restaurant with a particularly good meal; discussions of rationing fresh water, mending sails, and cleaning the boat.

But the log also details moments of high spirits and adventure, much of it centered on sailing, swimming, meeting new friends, exploring countless islands, and gathering the fruits of the land and sea, which the couple tried to live on as much as possible. By early January, *Just Dandy* had sailed into the waters of Exuma, a district of the Bahamas, consisting of more than 365 islands, also called cays.

On January 3, they took the dinghy out for a swim, dropping Gordon a half mile from the boat. As he swam back, he was tailed by a five-foot shark that followed him all the way. Later, after sailing some more, he writes: "This is why I came. LOVE IT!"

On January 22 at Highbourne Cay, Gordon speared a jackfish. As he hauled it in, a moray eel sprung out of a crevice and snatched it off his spear. Luckily, his spearfishing friend John got seven gray snapper at a reef, so they had a cookout. Gordon cooked the fish in beer and made a skillet of cornbread.

"We built a nice fire on the high hill and first fried the fritters and then had the fish, cornbread, salad and spuds," he writes. "We had a great time and everyone was stuffed…We swapped a lot of great stories and some songs. It was a super nice night and we could see lightning way off to the east."

On the 27th, after another day of successful reef fishing, Gordon made a fish pie—"A lot of work, but worth the effort." That night he decided to sleep outside on deck: "It was a great night and the stars were out by the millions."

The next day there was more fishing and eating with newfound friends, John and Kim. The day's take included a four-pound grouper, two queen triggers, and three smaller fish. Gordon also gathered conch, and for dinner there was broiled fish, chowder, and conch fritters. "We had a super time and everyone was happy," he writes.

Throughout these months, Gordon and Carol became part of a close-knit shoal of sailors who anchored together, watched each other's backs, and shared food, drink, supplies, stories, songs, weed, adventures, and good times with each other.

Gordon looks like he might have been able to pull up anchor and live this way indefinitely. In fact, in several April log entries, he writes of seriously considering an offer to stay in the islands and serve as a caretaker for a house located in Little Harbor. This decision-making process appears to have caused more conflict between the couple, and Gordon alludes to a "compromise" without providing details.

Since Carol had ceased to write in the log and declined to be interviewed, it must be surmised that she, perhaps, yearned for the comforts of home—or at least of dry land. Speaking years afterward, Gordon's sister Margo described the voyage (and the marriage) in a different light.

"She (Carol) was scared out of her mind—it was more than she could handle," she recalled. "That was not a big boat for such a voyage. I can't even imagine."

Gordon and Carol had a particularly bad scare near Rolleville on the sail between Lee Stocking Island and George Town.

"We got to Rolleville and anchored, but there was a bad swell, so we decided not to stay," Gordon writes. That would turn out to be an understatement. As they followed another boat to a cut between two islands, they were greeted by 200 yards of white water. As the first boat attempted to "buck the waves," it was nearly thrown over backward.

Gordon tried another cut and made it through, but then the wind picked up and he realized he had too much sail with his main sail, but he could not put up the jib, since he would not be able to sail windward. The best option at that point would have been to motor, but they were out of gas.

So they tacked back and forth as a novice skier facing a steep slope might shush back and forth, taking five hours to go fourteen miles. When they made it to a safe harbor, there was hardly room to drop anchor with so many boats waiting out the storm.

"Carol lost control and fell apart," Gordon writes. "I felt bad that I put her through that."

As bad as he may have felt, he loved sailing in any kind of weather and would have taken more risks on open water if he had been sailing alone. Not long after this episode, he writes: "I wish I could sail this boat the way I wanted to. But with Carol that is not possible."

Years later, as he aged and grew ill, depending on others for the first time, Gordon admitted to Nancy that as a young man he had been somewhat selfish, self-absorbed, and not necessarily the ideal partner in a relationship. The sailing obsession appears to be his, with Carol supporting his dream. His sister Margo echoes that theme.

"Gord loved sailing and he didn't care about a family. His priorities were more sailing than wanting to be home," Margo said. "He could make anything work, but that was him—he was not always thinking of the woman's side."

Throughout the voyage, while at anchor, Gordon would often take off alone in the dinghy or swim ashore to spend hours alone or making new friends without Carol, exploring, running, and sometimes biking, if he could borrow or rent one. Invariably, he would bring along his pipe.

His pot-smoking habit was a daily one and almost caused his arrest in Nassau, where police confiscated one pipe but could not find the stash he had discarded.

The arguments continued throughout, and Gordon mentions them frequently without providing much context or introspection. But they plugged along until mid-May, when job commitments forced them to cut the trip short. The original plan (Gordon's no doubt) had been to sail back up along the Eastern Seaboard and tow the boat home from an East Coast state. Instead, they sailed back up through the Intracoastal along the coast of Florida and the Gulf, Gordon noting his disappointment with leaving the islands behind and being back in US waters. They hired a towing company to tow the boat home from Atlanta. While Carol rode in the truck, he stayed back in the swaying boat.

In the back of the notebook of the second sailing log, there is an unsent letter addressed to "Kim, Beth, and the boys," sailing friends they had made in the Bahamas. In the letter, Gordon yearns to be back out on the water, though painting his and Carol's homecoming in a positive light. But this was not to last. The last two words in the sailing log capture Gordon's probable state of mind and mood: "Damn Xerox!"

IN THE PRE-VOYAGE interview with the *Holland Sentinel*, "there was only one area of concern that (Gordon) voiced about his trip. 'That is the biggest question. Will we be able to get along?'"

Unfortunately, his words proved prophetic. The couple's triumphant return was dampened by the realization that their marriage was damaged beyond repair. Gordon resumed working for Xerox, and when he had the opportunity within the next year, he bid for a new territory along the lakeshore several hours north of Holland, where he would relocate, without Carol, to the remote Lake Michigan town of Pentwater.

There, high atop a hill overlooking Pentwater Lake, he would, over the years, construct an idiosyncratic abode that manifested the essence of Gordon: exposed to the west wind, looking off to the horizon, charming, humble, rough-hewn, and slightly askew.

6

The Swimmer:
The Dutch Masters

*"These years were so fulfilling that the loss of my own mojo
was much easier to accept."*

—FRED NELIS

WHILE FRED WAS BECOMING an All-American at Kalamazoo College, with plans to pursue teaching and coaching following graduation, Fred Sr. was looking for an investment with staying power that he could pass on to the next generation of Nelises.

Having sold his share of Nelis' Dutch Village to his brother Harry in 1974, he had the capital. All he needed now was the right opportunity. In his daily reading of the *Wall Street Journal,* he came across what seemed like the perfect fit. Nothing could have more staying power than industrial vises, which, at the risk of being obvious, is what they are built to provide.

Yost Vises was founded in 1908 in Meadville, Pennsylvania, by the G. W. Yost Family. In the 1960s, the company was purchased and relocated to Muskegon, Michigan, about forty miles north along the lakeshore from Holland.

Fred Sr. made the decision to purchase the barely functioning factory in March 1979 and move it to Holland. There were a handful of employees in place, but the business was run by an absentee owner with a large stack of accounts payable.

Fred Sr. set about getting the business's books in order, and before Fred knew it, his teaching and coaching dreams once again were on hold as he gradually began devoting himself full-time to the new family venture.

At about the time Gordon was gallivanting around the sunlit Caribbean, Fred was spending twelve-hour days hunkered down in a dark factory and warehouse trying to make Yost Vises a profitable venture.

"Being relentless is the only business model I know," Fred recalled. "We have lost battles, but outlasted all our competitors. Not bragging, just fact."

The early years were not without their struggles, however. Government contracts through the US General Services Administration (GSA) kept the operation afloat through the lean, early years, when Fred worked alongside his father, brother Kevin, and one employee in a hot warehouse full of metal shavings and deafening machinery to produce, pack, load, and ship their product.

The GSA's biggest customer was the US Department of Defense. However, as the US military footprint began shrinking in the late 1970s and early 1980s with the withdrawal from Vietnam and the closing of US Naval Base Subic Bay and other overseas bases, Yost began to see a shrinking demand for their product as military motor pools, repair shops, and machine shops closed their doors.

A move by the GSA to open its catalogue to other government agencies probably kept the Nelises from going out of business or having to sell the company.

"The losses of the DOD were made up by shipyards, the National Guard, and Warren Tank Command," Fred recalled. "At one time we outfitted a couple of aircraft carrier groups. Our biggest purchase order was for 2,000 vises going to one of these carrier groups."

By the mid-1980s, the GSA comprised about 80 percent of Yost Vises' accounts, providing much-needed stability. The company's name was even included in most GSA bid requests and specs, which called for "Yost or equivalent" in terms of quality.

"It was the mid-80s that was the watershed moment for us, that gave us the opportunity to have a real strong financial position," Fred recalled.

By the early nineties, Fred and Kevin were joined by younger brother Tom. During those years, it was common practice for Fred and his brothers to work Monday through Friday 7 a.m. to 5 p.m., then come back after dinner from 7–10 p.m., and work a half day on Saturday.

"Over three years we aggressively pursued tool contracts and were fortunate enough to be awarded contracts that captured our entire line of products," he added. "We had back-to-back-to-back financial success."

With Fred's family growing to include four daughters, and with the health challenges that would confront the family in the 1990s, the financial stability was welcome. Yet, there was something missing.

"The career I thought I always wanted was to be a swim coach," Fred recalled.

Throughout the years he had dipped his toes in the water of coaching on a couple of occasions. He had his first taste of coaching during college, when he worked with a summer AAU (Amateur Athletic Union) program in Kalamazoo called the Y Kats, writing daily workouts, keeping youth swimmers focused on training, and coaching weekend swim meets.

By the late 1980s and early 1990s, when their daughters became old enough to compete, Fred and Jean helped salvage the township recreational swimming program, which was on the verge of closing for lack of a coach.

"Kelly and Heather were already involved in the program, so one of us needed to be there to drive the kids to and home from practice anyway," Fred recalled.

"I asked parents to join me on the deck assisting with coaching and technique instruction," he said. "This proved to be a very rewarding experience for me and also for the parents."

Somewhere along the way, he developed a regimen for training and competing that he dubbed "The Four F's" (Fun, Friends, Food, and Fitness), which encompasses not only his approach to the sport that is his passion, but along with a fifth F (Faith) helps to provide a guide to the other areas of his life.

Five years after Fred's diagnosis of idiopathic cardiomyopathy, in 1999, the communities within the Holland Public School District created a municipal authority to build the gorgeous, state-of-the art Holland Community Aquatic Center.

"It wasn't just a 50-meter, 750,000-gallon pool, but a jewel of the community," Fred said.

This "jewel," which would become Fred's home away from home, totals 86,745 square feet on two city blocks in central Holland, immediately adjacent to Holland Hospital, and contains competition, leisure, therapy, and instructional pools, as well as a fitness center, meeting rooms, and other amenities.

An array of programs for junior and high school swimmers were initiated or ramped up, but Fred and others noted a lack of opportunities for adult swimmers. The solution was an evening United States Masters Swimming workout for adults with a variety of skill levels, ranging from an interest in fitness all the way to competing at the annual US Masters Swimming Nationals.

Despite his ongoing health battles, Fred took on the challenge of leading this program, eventually becoming vice chair and then chair of the Michigan Region of US Masters Swimming.

In a dozen years of coaching, leading up to Fred's LVAD and eventual transplant, the "Dutch Masters," as they came to be called, won four state championships, and individual team members captured dozens of high point awards. As each success mounted, the club's reputation grew and new members clamored to join. Many agree that as a "Water Whisperer," Fred had found his true calling.

"In the swimming community, he is kind of a connector," said Steve Van Wylen, a thoracic and general surgeon who knows Fred about as well as anyone. Van Wylen competed against Fred in high school, swam for him on the Dutch Masters, and has served as his swim practice partner for many years.

"He's got a nice way of encouraging people of all types of abilities and styles," he added. "I've seen him take a complete stranger who comes to the pool and give him a couple of pointers to make him swim better."

"I just about drowned that first month, but Fred kept urging me from the pool deck to keep going," said Natalie Dykstra, a member of the Dutch Masters. "I learned that excuses just get in the way of life and that there was power in just getting in the water. Even now, I bring whatever difficulty I'm facing to the pool. Moving my body through water clarifies things for me—and I learned that first from being on Fred's Masters swim team. I'm forever grateful."

Fred's training philosophy was somewhat unusual for hardcore adult swimmers. Swimming is considered by some to be a boring solitary activity. Fred considers it, instead, to be a thinking sport, in which one needs to concentrate on the small details of the task at hand—the next breath and the next stroke. And to ensure freshness, no two practices are ever exactly the same.

Steve Van Wylen recalls a training activity Fred devised called "The Dirty Dozens."

"There was almost always going to be something that was a break from the routine," Van Wylen said. "The Dirty Dozens were 50-yard swim intervals, and for each one the rest between swims was diminished. 'Don't burn the first one,' he would say. By the end you were hanging on to finish."

"Don't burn the first one of a set" is just one of Fred's many trademark mantras that teammates recall. Others include: "It's not how far you swim, it's how fast you swim far," "A fast start is no guarantee of a strong finish," "No better feeling than to reel in a sprinter," and everyone's favorite, "The shower is the best part of swimming."

Beyond the slogans, however, Fred is thoughtful, even philosophical about his sport. It becomes obvious that swimming is a form of reflection and meditation, and he credits the sport with teaching him the difference between fear and anticipation.

"To swim is to be honest with yourself," Fred says. "Fear immobilizes you. But when you swim competitively, you've got to go through the moment, not pass over it.

"You are standing there in your skinny little trunks and you know in a minute and a half it will be over one way or another," he adds. "And if you don't win, you go back and work out harder and try again. But I knew through swimming that eventually things work out, and that was my attitude toward my illness and the transplant.

"Boredom leads to fatigue, so creativity was paramount to my coaching philosophy," Fred recalls. And his promise to all was that if he couldn't complete the workout, then they wouldn't have to either. For many years, not completing a workout was never a consideration. For despite his love of teaching, Fred remained a fierce competitor.

"He would come into the workouts and expect to keep up," said Masters Swimmer Janet Jasker. "He was very competitive. It would bother him if certain people beat him. He wanted to get the time he wanted."

However, as his illness progressed and he grew closer to the necessity of a transplant, others noticed a gradual change.

"Fred has changed over the years," said Bob Insalaco, another member of the team. "When I first met him it was all about winning when swimming. I think he has evolved to where he realizes winning would be nice, but just to be able to swim is everything."

"Typically he had more strength and speed and endurance than I did in the pool," Steve Van Wylen recalled. "All of a sudden we were swimming evenly and he was breathing heavier than I. His heart was going downhill again—and he knew it."

"Sometimes he wasn't feeling too well and would be leaning up against the pole," Janet Jasker said. "But he would always make the time to come and coach us."

Fred spent countless volunteer hours over the years on behalf of this labor of love.

"Coaching Masters was important for me because I could watch the development and continued strong performances of team members, all the while knowing my competitive days were numbered," Fred recalls. "Athletes know when *that* time has come and I was very aware of my own descending spiral. At least I could live through the team's successes.

"The greatest compliment I received was someone saying, 'I never thought I could do that,'" he adds. "Who needs money when you witness such a moment?"

Through his involvement in the Dutch Masters, Fred found a colleague on the other side of the state who would serve as an ally in developing Masters Swimming programs in Michigan, and who eventually would become a mentor.

Ralph Davis, 71, of Brighton, is the retired CFO of Federal-Mogul Corporation, a manufacturer and supplier of automotive, commercial, aerospace, marine, rail and off-road vehicle products. Like Fred, he is Midwest born-and-bred, a conservative with a strong work ethic, and a family man married to wife Bonnie, a pilot, for 52 years, with three daughters and five grandchildren. Both are men of faith with a lengthy history of donating time to religious and charitable organizations, strong civic involvement and giving back to the community.

Like Fred he was also an athlete who maintained himself in good physical condition as a competitive swimmer, running, in addition, up to thirty-five miles per week.

In 2005, Davis suffered atrial fibrillation, an irregular heartbeat caused by the abnormal firing of electrical impulses. Following several rounds of cardioversion therapy to restart the heart over the next year, he was eventually fitted with a pacemaker and defibrillator. After an adverse reaction to antibiotics created a pulmonary embolism, his heart began to fail, and on February 11, 2006, he received a heart transplant from an 18-year-old donor.

"Everyone who gets a transplant remembers their birthdays," Davis said. "I always celebrate that as a second birthday. It is your second opportunity for a gift of life.

When it came time for Fred to consider the inevitability of LVAD and transplant, Ralph Davis was a close friend who could understand the incredible mix of feelings involved and provide greatly appreciated counsel.

A VAD (ventricular assist device) is an electromechanical device, implanted in the chest, for improving cardiac circulation, used to replace or assist the function of a failing heart. VADs are designed to assist either the right ventricle (RVAD), the left ventricle (LVAD), or both ventricles (BiVAD).

As his ejection fraction numbers worsened, Davis advised a hesitant Fred to get on the list for an LVAD. Later, when he began doing better with his LVAD, Fred called to say he wasn't sure if he wanted to be listed for transplant.

"I told him I know you feel great on the LVAD, but you just won't believe how great you will feel after you get your transplant," Davis recalled. "I just wanted to give him confidence that all will be well come June 18, 2014.

"Fred is just one of those people who are the salt of the earth," Davis said. "He is a good person who would be willing to help anyone who was down and out or in need."

Fred is a man of contradictions—an enthusiastic and passionate teacher, a gifted athlete, and a fierce competitor determined to beat his rivals in sport or business, yet someone willing to give a stranger the shirt off his back.

Of course Fred's entire approach to life can't be boiled down to a simple slogan like his swimming regimen of "The Four F's." But he does enjoy devising such slogans, as well as creating T-shirts and nicknames for all occasions.

He seems to have been born with a smile on his face, yet he binds his happiness to a yoke of duty and a mantle of hard work, albeit one inscribed by practical jokers.

All of it comes to the fore in the Dutch Masters, which, in many ways, is the culmination of Fred's life's work—the arena where he could share the hard-won knowledge of a lifetime of cold morning practices and an urgency to reach and go farther, faster, smoother, better than ever before.

7

The Sailor:
The Gordwardian Knot

Gordon on sailing in a storm: "Either you get hit by lightning or you don't. If you get hit by lightning, either you live or you don't. And in any case, you have a great story to tell."

(As quoted by JOE CLARK)

Gordon on storytelling: "Never let the truth get in the way of a good story."

(As quoted by JOHN VANDE BUNTE)

DESPITE THE REGRET of his failed marriage, life continued as a grand adventure for Gordon.

A few years after his Bahamas sailing adventure, Gordon cooked up a new invention that fused sailing with his other great love, biking. By this time he was something of a local celebrity and repeatedly made the headlines of the *Ludington Daily News*:

It takes only a few moments for Pentwater's Gordon Veldman to hook his homemade kayak trailer to his 12-speed bicycle and be off on a day of fun and relaxation.

Gordon likes to bike, thinks boating of all kinds is just about tops, and doesn't care so much for automobiles. So, when he wants to get away from it all on an afternoon or weekend, he hitches a kayak to his 12-speed bicycle and away he goes.

'I'm a biker, but most of all I love the water,' he said. 'Water is the last endeavor of pure nature in this world.'

"Gordon would bike 60, 70, 80 miles at a time," said Pentwater friend Dave Spitler. "He loved to bike early morning and late evening. Sometimes he'd ride all night."

In addition to sailing and biking, Gordon was an avid runner from his US Army days all the way to his Alpha-1 diagnosis. He jogged daily around Pentwater Lake, clocking his times and running in the annual Lakestride Half Marathon. He reveled in the outdoors, and in an awesome level of physical fitness that allowed him to do virtually anything he wanted. In short, as his friends will attest, before Alpha-1 laid him low, he was always on the go.

His restless energy is perhaps best exemplified by the rope swing that for many years hung looped around the railings of his deck overlooking Pentwater Lake. The fulcrum end was tied to the overhanging limb of a huge oak, and when mounted, the contraption swung out from the deck to the sheer drop-off on the west side of Gordon's property. In the midst of an animated deckside conversation or perhaps even during dinner, Gordon would occasionally slide his foot into the loop and swing out into the void for a momentary thrill before dismounting and resuming his conversation in mid-sentence.

Gordon has too many friends to count, but they can be roughly broken down into a few periods of his adult life, including his sailing friends from Holland, Michigan, where he lived throughout the 1970s and into the early 1980s; his Pentwater, Michigan, friends, where he has lived since the early 1980s; and those friends scattered throughout the world whom he tries to visit and keep in touch with as much as he can.

But Gordon is the ultimate extrovert and can make friends anywhere. He also had a number of relationships and romantic entanglements throughout the 1980s, following his divorce from Carol. But he finally found new love with second wife, Beverly Fogarty, a Ludington, Michigan, native, whom he married in 1989 and stayed with for nearly 20 years.

"Gordon had this childlike sense of wonder," Fogarty says. "One of the things we enjoyed doing was walking in the woods and watching sunsets. He never tired of sunsets. It was as if every sunset was a new thing. He made me see things in a new way."

One of the things that impressed her was the trapeze Gordon had rigged up in the vaulted ceiling of his living room.

"On our first date he invited me to his house and made me dinner," she recalls. "Of course I noticed the rope swing off the deck and the trapeze in the house. Of course I immediately had to try it," she says. "And every once in a while he would get up there and swing from his knees."

Another was the realization that they shared a fascination with the books of Richard Halliburton.

"The thing that struck me most was that he had a copy of *Richard Halliburton's Book of Marvels*," Beverly says. "That book was pivotal for me as a kid. I used to check it out of the library every other week."

Halliburton, an American traveler, adventurer, and author, captivated readers of the 1920s and 1930s with his daring adventures, chronicled in the newsreels and in a series of books that became best sellers.

In his first book, 1925's *The Royal Road to Romance*, the 25-year-old Halliburton, only three years removed from Princeton, sets forth his agenda: "Let those who wish have their respectability," he writes. "I wanted freedom, freedom to indulge in whatever caprice struck my fancy, freedom to search in the farthermost corners of the earth for the beautiful, the joyous and the romantic."

In 1939, while attempting to sail a Chinese junk from Hong Kong to San Francisco, he was lost at sea and presumed drowned. It is no wonder that he is a favorite of Gordon's. And in Beverly, Gordon had found a kindred spirit with the same free-spirited willingness to say "yes" to adventure.

Following graduation from Western Michigan University in 1972 with a bachelor's degree in English and sociology and a master's in counseling, Beverly and a friend took off for Southern California, sleeping on a friend's brother's sofa until they found work in Los Angeles as cocktail waitresses and go-go dancers.

After a few months of saving up their tips, they set off with $450 and backpacked for months throughout Mexico and Central and South America, eventually hitchhiking back to LA from Mexico City. The two attractive young women had no trouble obtaining rides.

"We got a lot of freebies too," she recalled. "A free flight and free ride on a tugboat down the Amazon."

Upon her return Beverly accepted a job as a counselor at a Mason County school district. Mutual friends, intuiting that the two could hit it off, conspired for Beverly and Gordon to meet. Together, the couple, unencumbered by children, took off on too many adventures to recount, sailing the San Blas Islands of Panama, spending a Christmas in Tahiti, and another in New Zealand in the early 1990s that came to be known as the "Miracle of the Nativity."

On that particular Christmas Eve, Gordon and Beverly attempted to spend the holiday with their friends Greg and Barb Siewert in New Zealand. They rented a car but got lost in the bush trying to find their friends' home.

Like most good stories, this is a pre-cellphone-era story, which may partly explain Gordon's antipathy toward cellphones. They have ruined many a fine potential story as well as many a fine movie plot, and he continues to carry a flip phone to this day.

The Siewerts waited and waited, with no word, for the Veldmans to arrive, putting their Christmas Eve on hold until they were forced to carry on and celebrate without the wayward couple.

Meanwhile, a kind-hearted Kiwi farming couple put Gordon and Beverly up for the night, when they could finally go no farther. The accommodations were rustic, not unlike the place where the Christ child entered the world—an old trailer in an overgrown sheep pasture.

"They woke up on Christmas morning to the sound of the sheep scratching their backs against the trailer," said Greg Siewert. "It was almost a manger scene."

WITH GORDON'S SENSE of adventure in mind, several of his friends have come to refer to his unique (some might say "cockeyed") point of view as "Gordwardian Theories" or "The Gordwardian Way." Other friends, unfamiliar with the term, nonetheless nod in immediate understanding when it is explained.

Although a distinguishing factor of the Gordwardian Way is that of improvisation and an avoidance of categories, these loose strands of unenumerated philosophy can be grouped together in a number of different ways:

ENTHUSIASM AND A SENSE OF WONDER AND CURIOSITY

Gordon returned to the Bahamas for several weeks in early 1996 to join his friend Don McDonald, who was sailing a boat he had crafted by hand.

In his sailing log, McDonald notes the horrendous weather that made sailing all but impossible the first few weeks of 1996. On January 17, he writes "I call Gord, the man with no negatives. He reassured me good weather will be there when he arrives. I love that character and can't wait for his arrival."

True to form, the arrival of Gordon's sunny disposition coincided with a change in the weather, and they set off sailing immediately. Gordon found that some things had changed in the decade and half since his last visit. Sailing between Little Bell Island and Staniel Cay, Gord notes in the log that there is now a $500 fine for spearfishing and the taking of conch. The log also notes an inundation of "Richie Rich" yachts that were not as ubiquitous in days gone by.

But Gordon could still wax lyrical about the sights, sounds and sensations of the sea. Sailing near Hoffman's Cay on the 31st, he writes:

We floated over a 5 ft. deep sandy bottom in the moonlight. This was one of the greatest experiences I have ever had on a boat. Four porpoise were swimming with us for a spell. One surfaced just behind us and I saw its eye shine bright blue for about a half second...We could see starfish, sponges, conch grass, everything as it slid by under our hulls.

Beverly has already mentioned Gordon's fascination with sunsets, but, as noted, his appreciation of nature does not stop with the setting of the sun.

"Gordon took us out in a metal rowboat, in November, to see the stars," said John Vande Bunte. "The stars were amazing."

The frozen lakes of a Michigan winter are also no deterrent to his quest to see, experience and marvel at the wonders of nature. Another endeavor that fused Gordon's love of nature, fitness and gadgetry was an ice sailboat that he constructed in the early 1990s. This invention led to another write-up in the *Ludington Daily News*, which described him as "a fan of 'free fun,' meaning non-mechanically powered recreation such as sailing—on water or ice—skating, and bicycling...he keeps a close watch on ice conditions. Some years, the right conditions for ice sailing may last for a day—or less."

Sometimes, however, Gordon's sense of wonder skates out onto the thin ice of the next category.

ZEST FOR LIFE (WITH A CERTAIN AMOUNT OF FEARLESSNESS, RECKLESSNESS AND RISK-TAKING)

John Vande Bunte tells the story of the time that he, Gordon, and Steve Wolff, all big men well over six feet tall, went ice skating on the pond near Gordon's Pentwater home.

"Gordon would ice skate on the thin ice with a 12-foot pole in case he fell through," Vande Bunte recalled. "All of a sudden, you could see the ice collapse and Steve and I scrambled for shore. Gord stayed on the ice. Gord is out there going, 'Oh that ice is safe.'"

Another Pentwater friend, the photographer Joe Clark, recalls Gordon's words the first time the two sailed together in a Lake Michigan storm.

"Either you get hit by lightning or you don't," Clark recalled. "If you get hit by lightning, either you live or you don't. And in any case, you have a great story to tell."

"I remember running into Gord sailing in some out-of-the-way channel naked or in his tighty-whiteys," John Vande Bunte recalled. "He never insured his boat, because, why would he? If things are going to happen, they are going to happen."

"Gordon would never say no to an escapade," said Heide Kenjorski. "If he doesn't have a prior commitment, he is there."

Gordon's favorite sailing destination on the Great Lakes is the North Channel, a pristine wilderness stretching some 160 nautical miles along the north shore of Lake Huron, considered by many to be some of the finest freshwater sailing in the world. Despite the lure of its clear waters, hundreds of islands, and hidden anchorages, sailing the North Channel is not for the faint of heart. Water depths can vary considerably and, because of the remoteness of the region, provisions, fuel, and help in case of an emergency may be difficult to come by.

Gordon and Beverly sailed the North Channel many times, often in the company of Dave and Chrissie Hall, sailing friends from Ludington. Dave Hall recalled that Gordon, ever the gregarious extrovert, would often intentionally leave his boat ladder in the water to invite conversation from other sailors.

"Before we met Gordon and Beverly, we heard people talk about them as if they were deities," Dave Hall said.

"There is a narrow passage in the North Channel through the Benjamin Islands that Gordon referred to as 'The Garage,'" said Chrissie Hall. "Gordon could navigate that channel blindfolded."

"It is not recommended to sail through The Slot, which is two very narrow cliffs about 50 feet wide," said Dave Hall. "Gordon has a photo of himself jumping naked off one of the 60-foot cliffs. He made multiple copies for all of his sailing friends, who would be sure to recognize the landmark."

Dave also remembers a time in the North Channel when Gordon and Beverly went in search of wild blueberries and came across the scat of a large animal. Later, as the two couples sat on the decks of their boats enjoying blueberry pancakes, they sailed past a pair of gigantic moose.

"They were great pancakes," Dave recalled.

A SENSE OF CELEBRATION

Gordon and Beverly became well-known in the Pentwater-Ludington area for their themed parties, which included solstice parties, Hawaiian luaus, and numerous other excuses for fun and revelry:

When Gordon was downsized into an early retirement from Xerox in his early fifties, Beverly threw a "Bring Gordon a Project to Keep Him Busy" party in honor of his birthday and his retirement. One guest broke a toilet into 1,000 pieces, boxed them up and presented them to Gordon along with a bottle of glue.

When the couple made their final payment on an adjoining property they were particularly happy to purchase, they celebrated by hosting a "Fence-Down Party." The mission of the 20–30 assembled guests was to try to topple the fence that sat in the way of their view of Pentwater Lake.

At a "Tacky Party" the couple hosted, Beverly served jugged wine, pigs in a blanket and Spam, while Gordon vacuumed in the middle of the party and threatened to give a slide show presentation of his vacation.

During the early 1990s, Beverly and two friends took belly dancing classes. A friend of Gordon's who was celebrating a birthday was led to believe that, as a present, he would be entertained by three lovely female belly dancers. As the birthday boy waited in delighted anticipation, a signal was given, an air of exotic Mediterranean music wafted through the house and the clicking of castanets drew closer. When those assembled could barely stand another moment's wait, down the stairs came two huge bearded men in full belly-dancing regalia: Gordon and another large, hirsute friend.

SHARING THE GIFT OF FRIENDSHIP

Greg and Barb Siewert are part of the old Holland sailing gang. Through Greg's work in the sailing industry as a boat designer, they have known many ports of call as home, including Charleston, San Diego, Seattle and as mentioned, New Zealand.

"Gordon is one of the few friends who has visited us in every location," said Greg Siewert. "He is a very loyal friend. In fact, we used to joke about unpacking the boxes quickly when we moved so there would be room for him to sleep."

As evidenced by the plethora of anecdotes, friendship and the sharing of experiences with friends may well be the most important undertaking of Gordon's life. As the ultimate extrovert, his euphoric peak experiences, whether sunsets, the eye of a surfacing porpoise, or jumping naked from a cliff, carry added significance when shared with friends.

In fact, the sharing of Fred and Gordon's transplant experience with the media and the general public, as well as the writing of this book, can trace their roots to that impulse.

"When the shared transplant with Fred happened, I thought this is so cool, it can't just be a secret story between two old guys," Gordon recalled.

"You see, having a shared experience or a memory with someone I hold dear improves and expands it by not just 100, but 1,000 percent," he added.

SELF-RELIANCE AND STICK-TO-IT-NESS

Gordon's skill with machinery, engineering, and carpentry, interest in scientific inquiry, and enthusiasm for gadgets has come in handy (and saved the day) on numerous occasions.

As Beverly has shared, it served him well in his professional life at Xerox and seems to be an innate ability, because Gordon lacks any formal mechanical and engineering training.

"You have to keep Gordon busy," Barb Siewert recalled. "I woke up one morning in San Diego, and there he was on the floor fixing my vacuum cleaner.

"I still have that same vacuum cleaner," she added.

"He also fixed my miter saw on that trip," Greg Siewert recalled.

Gordon's friend Dave Spitler is a licensed professional contractor and former industrial arts professor at Central Michigan University.

"Gordon has no construction knowledge, but he looks at things from a unique perspective and it allows him to do some rather bizarre, but impressive projects," said Spitler. "The way he goes about things is just unique. He is a very bright guy and he has a lot of stick-to-it-ness.

"For example, if he saw a bunch of glass he might get the idea to build a greenhouse," Spitler added.

"I would ask him, 'How did you manage to get the design for a greenhouse?' 'Well, I decided to use these metal pieces so they wouldn't move so much and break the glass,' and I'd say 'that's exactly what you need to do.'

"We are very alike because we both like to see how things work," he added. "We have had a lot of discussions about that kind of stuff that would bore most people out of their minds."

Gordon may be a fascinating character, but like all of us, he is far from perfect.

Beverly says that Gordon's sense of wonder is a double-edged sword.

"Having that childlike sense of wonder also made him somewhat childish," she said. "In our marriage, he was selfish—always doing what he wanted.

"One of the bones of contention is that I'm an avid reader and he always wanted to be out doing things," she added. "He would be mad when he'd walk through the house and see me reading.

"The biggest problem we had was I was 40 when we got married, I had sisters I was close to, and he really resented any time I spent away from him," she said. "It was kind of an old-school feeling like his parents' marriage where they did everything together."

Beverly said that Gordon's fascination with the way things work did not apply to the workings of his own mind or to their relationship.

"He wasn't very introspective," she said. "He is very much an extrovert and could be around people 24/7. It just amazes me. I'm energized by being alone.

"I dragged us off to marriage counseling one time," Beverly said. "A fabulous woman in Muskegon. 'Gordon,' she said, 'you are a fascinating man, but I don't want you to waste your money.' He understood the theory but was not in touch with the underlying feelings.

"I think that the Alpha-1 diagnosis served as a great life lesson for him," she said. "Coming down with a grave illness made it much easier for him to deal with the pain and sadness of others."

8

The Swimmer: Dead Man's Float

Dead Man's Float: *Also known as the jellyfish or survival float, one of the most important skills for swimmers to learn, since it can help you survive in the water.*

IN 1994, Fred began noticing some inexplicable changes in his health. His swim times were slower. Often he couldn't catch his breath. When he lay down, his breathing worsened, to the point where he was gurgling. He took to sleeping on three pillows just so he could breathe.

It seemed insane. He was 38 years old and in prime physical shape. He didn't just swim; as he always said, he trained. Later his doctors would describe him as being in the "elite" category of athletes. So how could a competitive swimmer of his caliber suddenly experience such a drastic deterioration in physical stamina?

Finally, Jean insisted that it was time to take action. Like many men, Fred had preferred to ignore his symptoms, trying to convince himself he could tough it out. But he was finally bewildered and miserable enough to capitulate to reality. They drove to the Holland Hospital ER, where, after extensive testing, he received a diagnosis that sent him reeling: idiopathic cardiomyopathy.

"Idiopathic cardiomyopathy is essentially heart failure," said Fred. "It's what old folks die of." The idiopathic part of the disease essentially means "of unknown origin." The most probable explanation is a virus. Even though Fred's mother had cardiomyopathy herself, the disease has not been shown to be genetic.

"It was a shock, because I was very fit—swimming was my life," he said. "I swam on Monday and was diagnosed on Friday." To make matters worse, Fred and Jean received the news from a physician whose bedside manner was not exactly his strong suit. They now laughingly refer to "Dr. Frank and Earnest," who breezed into their room and delivered the news as matter-of-factly as if providing a weather report. But at the time it was no joke.

"The doctor came in, spent about five minutes with us, and said, 'Oh by the way, you have a 15 percent chance of recovery or you'll need a heart transplant,' and then left," recalled Fred. "Needless to say, we were stunned." Fred refers to the night he received the news as a double-edged sword.

"On the one hand, the news was terrible and this doctor was the first of many to not give me a chance," Fred recalled. "But the athlete in me took it as a challenge: 'Want to bet?' The heart is a muscle that has been injured. Like any muscle, it can be strengthened."

Tests revealed a dangerously low ejection fraction. EF, as it's called, is a measurement of the percentage of blood leaving the heart each time it contracts. During each heartbeat cycle, the heart contracts and relaxes. When the heart contracts, it ejects blood from the two pumping chambers (ventricles). When the heart relaxes, the ventricles refill with blood. No matter how forceful the contraction, it doesn't empty all of the blood out of a ventricle. The term "ejection fraction" refers to the percentage of blood that's pumped out of a filled ventricle with each heartbeat.

Because the left ventricle is the heart's main pumping chamber, ejection fraction is usually measured only in the left ventricle (LV). An LV ejection fraction of 55 percent or higher is considered normal. An LV ejection fraction of 30 percent or lower is considered dangerous.

Fred's EF was 10 percent. His heart was so compromised that it was astonishing he hadn't suffered cardiac arrest. His chest was filled with fluid. It was only because of his superior fitness level that he'd been able to maintain activity as long as he had.

Dr. Steve Van Wylen remembers seeing Fred and Jean in the hospital the morning of Fred's fateful diagnosis, while on duty as a thoracic and general surgeon. In the days prior to electronic medical records, patient information was sometimes kept on a private whiteboard where physicians could check room numbers and other patient information while making rounds.

"I'm checking the whiteboard and I see 'F. Nelis,' and I think, 'What in the world would Fred be doing in the ICU?'" Van Wylen recalled. "I popped my head in the door and there was Fred. I could see Jean sitting beside him. Her eyes were red and she had been crying.

"I asked Fred, 'What are you doing here?' and Fred smiles at me and says, 'It's nothing.' I looked at Jean and could tell it was something far more ominous than Fred was letting on." Fortunately, the fluid could be dealt with. Fred was released from Holland Hospital after four days. Eight pounds of fluid had been drained with the help of powerful diuretics. Fred went home with prescriptions for a half-dozen medications. It was a new experience.

"With the exception of an occasional mixed drink and a couple of beers a week, I never took any medication," Fred said. "Now I had prescriptions for hypertension and was taking half a dozen pills a day." But the meds were only going to stabilize him, not cure him. Soon after his discharge, Fred and Jean met with his internist, David Young, who sat them down for a literal heart-to-heart talk. Young's recommendation was sobering: begin preparations for the likelihood of a heart transplant.

At that time, there were two transplant centers in Michigan, at the University of Michigan Medical Center in Ann Arbor and at Henry Ford Hospital in Detroit. Young's preference was Henry Ford, and an appointment was made for late January. Meanwhile, Fred underwent a heart catheterization at Muskegon's Hackley Hospital. A wire inserted in the groin and going to the left ventricle recorded internal pressure and tissue samples. The test confirmed the diagnosis of a 10 percent ejection fraction. While everything went well, the possibility of re-opening the femoral artery was a serious problem. Fred definitely wasn't prepared for the fact that someone had to sit at his bedside for seven hours holding a sandbag on the wound site to ensure proper clotting.

When it was time to go to Henry Ford, Fred's parents drove him and Jean the three hours across the state to the consultation. It quickly became apparent to Fred that the doctors were not going to waste any time in getting straight to work.

"From the get-go, I had the impression that I might not be leaving Detroit any time soon," Fred said. Preparations were made with all the departments associated with transplants. Fred and his transplant coordinator visited infectious disease, pastoral care, surgery, psychiatry, and case management. Fred had an ultrasound, complete bloodwork, and finally a metabolic stress test.

"Being a kid from a small town, I was overwhelmed by the three grueling days of tests and consults," Fred said. "The psychological profile described me as a strong 'type A' personality. It also determined that I was in denial. I had no idea what the hell that was."

When asked by psychiatrists how he felt about having a transplant, he responded ruefully, "Like a vulture sitting on a fence post waiting for the injured animal to quit kicking so I could pick its bones without getting hurt."

After the meetings, blood draws, and various tests, it was time to finally meet the surgeon. This led to the only lighthearted moment Fred recalls. Upon entering the room, the surgeon, a young, confident man, asked who the patient was. Fred, Jean, and Mr. and Mrs. Nelis began to chuckle.

"When I introduced myself, the poor guy thought I was kidding," Fred said. "'You don't look like you need a transplant,' he said. Never judge a book by its cover!"

There was one more hurdle to go: the stress test, a guidance measure for unsupervised exercise based on effort level and heart rates.

The results provide valuable insight into the likelihood of developing an exercise-induced arrhythmia.

The test began with a gentle walk on a treadmill at a flat level. Every three minutes the speed and incline are increased. Fred's instructions were to proceed until exhaustion. Because his swim training had ended the first week of January, Fred felt his level of conditioning was fair at best, having had no meaningful exercise in the past month.

Fred walked on the treadmill, breathing into an apparatus that resembled a scuba mouthpiece, while two technicians kept track of his progress. Five, 10, 15 minutes passed. By this time he was running.

"The techs were relieved when I finally stopped at 18 minutes," he recalled. After the stress test results were evaluated, the cardiologist, Dr. Arlene Levine, met with Fred to discuss direction and options. She began with the issue of the 10 percent EF and the serious implications of such a poor pumping heart.

Fred fired a barrage of questions. Was there anything he could do to his heart to cause it further damage? Was there a chance it would improve? Since idiopathic cardiomyopathy has no connection to the coronary disease generally associated with heart failure, how likely was it that the heart muscle could be reconditioned? Finally, and top on his priority list, how long before he could start swimming again?

"By this time, I could tell that Dr. Levine was not only surprised but irritated at my attitude," Fred said. "Definitely denial!" When they came to the results of the stress test, Fred had no presumption of having done well. But to his astonishment, Dr. Levine dropped a bombshell. Never before in her experience had anyone with a 10 percent EF completed 18 minutes on the treadmill. Not only that, but no irregular or skipped beats were detected.

She congratulated Fred on his "superior level" of conditioning. It was all he needed to hear. He had only one question: "Can I do any further damage to my heart with exercise?" The answer then and thereafter was no. But it became apparent that Fred's idea of exercise and the doctors' were very different.

"My mind began to race," he recalled. "If I wanted to maintain that superior level, then I'll be back in the pool on Monday. Why wouldn't common sense prevail? I was where I was because of my swim training. I considered it the opposite of dangerous. My decades of discipline would assure compliance with the heart rate guidelines."

The three priorities in cardiac rehabilitation are diet, exercise, and medication. Fred had no trouble complying with the medical part. The diet aspect, however, was literally tough to swallow. He was told to follow a low fat/low sodium regimen. The only problem was that diet had nothing to do with his condition. He'd never had coronary artery disease, and his BMI, cholesterol, and triglycerides were all in the normal range.

When it came to exercise, Fred was like a bull pawing at the ground to get back into the ring, and locking horns with everyone else in the process. The results of the stress test put Fred at a maximum heart rate of 130 BPM for staying in the "safe" zone. Heart rate monitoring is a common practice for swimmers and is often used to evaluate training performance.

"If the doctors wanted me to stay under 130 BPM, fine," Fred said. "I could do what I enjoyed and be with my buddies at the pool." But apparently all exercise is not equal. In no time, Fred managed to antagonize his doctors and parents with his plan.

"Mom scolded me for most of the three-hour drive back to Holland," he recalled. "As a nurse and a thirty-year cardiomyopathy patient herself, she knew what she was talking about. I had better comply with the doctors' guidelines or else!"

As the tongue lashing went on, Fred felt his resolve crumbling. The following week, he began cardiac rehab classes. The rehab classes met three times a week, 50 minutes per session. While this schedule is too arduous for many patients, it didn't even make a dent in Fred's stamina.

"Here I was, taking a breather from my six to eight weekly hours of training and settling in for 'exercise,'" Fred said. "The whole idea seemed absurd."

It was time for a top-secret plan. Fred would do the monitored rehab class AND get back in the pool.

Things went smoothly until someone informed Fred's care team. Even though he was careful to stay within the recommended heart rate parameters, he was summoned posthaste back to Henry Ford and received another tongue lashing from his mother in the car.

"Then I got phase two from the doctors—something about not being safe should something happen," he said. "Maybe they thought I was swimming in the ocean." Downtrodden and tag-teamed from all sides, Fred relented—at least outwardly.

"The summer before he was diagnosed we had gotten a puppy," Jean Nelis recalled. "That spring he walked a lot with the dog. I'm sure he had depths of despair and some dark moments because we didn't know then if his heart was going to get better."

Fred worked through his despair toward a strengthened resolve. He told himself that just because he agreed to stay out of the pool didn't mean he'd given up. He made no bones about how unhappy he was at rehab. And his griping paid off. A woman on the rehab staff did some undercover work on her own and came up with a testing center at Presbyterian Hospital in Dallas that looked to be swimmer-friendly. She arranged a consult with, ironically, a doctor with the same last name as Fred's cardiologist at Henry Ford: Dr. Benjamin Levine.

Fred and Jean went to Dallas that June. Thanks to an endowment from H. Ross Perot, the facilities were brand new and featured the latest diagnostic tools for exercise evaluation, including one of only two high-velocity swimming flumes in the nation—the other located at the US Olympic Headquarters in Colorado Springs.

Dr. Levine administered all the tests himself. When he read Fred's latest EF, which had crested to 30 percent—high enough to take him off the transplant list for the time being—he could hardly contain his excitement.

"Fred, like many athletes, had a good sense of what he could and couldn't do," Dr. Levine recalled years later. "He knew that he could swim, but he was also a smart guy who didn't want to necessarily go against his doctor's orders and harm himself.

"That's why coming to Dallas was particularly validating," he added. "I wasn't particularly surprised by the results and neither was he."

Fred underwent the usual blood work and other tests. Dr. Levine had scheduled two metabolic stress tests, one on the treadmill and the other in the swimming flume, which was approximately 15 feet long and deep enough to prevent touching bottom. Both tests had exactly the same protocol—a 12-lead heart monitor and a scuba-type mouthpiece to record oxygen/carbon dioxide exchange.

"I was most excited about the flume," Fred said. "When the command was given to begin swimming, a stream of water shot out from the front of the tank. In a sense, you were like a salmon fighting to swim against the current of the river."

The speed of the flow was measured with a flow meter, and as the flow increased, so did the effort to maintain position. Hence the resistance-heart rate correlation was calculated exactly as if the patient were on a treadmill. Fred waited on pins and needles for the results that he hoped would end the drama with his Henry Ford physicians.

"The fear on the part of his physicians was two-fold; one was that swimming could raise the pressure in his heart too high and he would not be able to swim or he might develop pulmonary edema," Dr. Levine said. "And two, if he had a problem like arrhythmia, or if his heart stopped, he'd be in the water and he could drown."

To Fred's relief, and with a big smile on his face, Dr. Levine announced that he could find no medical reason that he shouldn't swim. All the data from the treadmill and the flume correlated exactly. The tests showed no arrhythmia with exercise, putting to rest concerns about his safety in the water.

"We were able to tell his doctors that swimming is the sport that Fred loves, and he can do it safely without hurting himself," Dr. Levine said.

"The world has changed since then," he added. Thanks to several landmark studies, today cardiologists recognize that exercise training can be vital for patients with heart failure.

"It reduces the risk of hospitalization and of mortality," Dr. Levine said. "Fred was ahead of his time."

Before Fred left Dallas, Dr. Levine put him on a beta blocker, a drug that was just coming into vogue. The drug slowed the heart and helped to develop a more powerful contraction. Unfortunately, while beta blockers have been a godsend to heart patients, slowing down the heart rate also means putting a governor on the upper limits of heart rate.

"I didn't quite understand why, if I had the OK to swim, I needed another medication," Fred said. "It took me awhile to come to grips with going 55 in a 70-mph speed zone."

Back at Henry Ford, Fred enjoyed the sweet taste of victory. The mood changed from "No!" to "Please be careful." After the doctors gave him the green light, training started in earnest. It was July and Fred set himself a goal to accomplish a workout he had done frequently prior to his diagnosis by October. It was a challenge he didn't know if he could meet. First, he wasn't sure there was enough time to get back in shape. Then the beta blockers presented an additional obstacle to swimming at the speed he needed to train at.

The October day finally arrived for Fred's self-defined "test of physical and mental toughness."

"I was doing this because if I could pull it off, I'd have the assurance that I'd be OK," Fred said. "With little fanfare and no witnesses, I completed ten x 200-yard swims on a three-minute interval. Totally spent, I climbed out of the pool and went home for a nap."

When Fred returned to Henry Ford in October for a checkup, he was surprised and delighted to learn that the transplant team had decided to ask him to return his beeper. His progress had been steady, and coming off a 10 percent ejection fraction to a consistent 30 percent qualified him for removal from transplant consideration. It would be his last visit; in December, Dr. Levine released him from her care.

Thanks to his insistence and self-advocacy (and some might add stubbornness), Fred had accomplished what many failed to believe possible. He had literally swum himself off the transplant list. Although he had not completely escaped danger, he had bought himself a significant amount of time.

It would be twelve years before new health problems descended, and old ones resurfaced.

9

The Sailor: Dead in the Water

The phrase "dead in the water" used to refer to sailing ships that stopped moving because the wind stopped blowing… It now refers to any floating vessel that can't propel itself because of an engine malfunction, damage, or lack of fuel.

STILL JOGGING IN 1997 at the age of 49, Gordon noticed something disturbing. His running times were getting slower. Soon afterward, he contracted double pneumonia following surgery for a knee fracture.

According to Gordon's recollection, it was supposed to be a 20-minute surgery that lasted three hours. In the middle of the surgery, the surgeon was called out to the ER and Gordon remained under general anesthesia until the surgeon returned.

"The next morning I couldn't breathe," Gordon said. "I had double pneumonia, and from then on, things got gradually worse."

Gradual was the operative word. Gordon's decline was steeper than Fred's, though a slow enough progression that he could deny what was happening to him.

"I was not proactive with my own health," he said. "I just hoped it would go away."

But by 2007, "it" had not. Instead, Gordon's breathing capacity had deteriorated to the point where Beverly took matters into her own hands. "We've got to find out what's going on with you," she insisted, and made an appointment with a pulmonologist.

The news wasn't good.

"You're in bad shape," he bluntly informed Gordon after the results of a blood test came back. "You have Alpha-1."

There is no cure for Alpha-1. The only available treatment that could possibly slow the progression of the disease and improve Gordon's lung capacity was a protein replacement gleaned from plasma. The doctor proposed starting Gordon on regular infusions. But Gordon, being Gordon, had other priorities.

"I was going on this sailing trip in four or five months, and I thought, it's silly to be starting on something that has to be done every couple of weeks," he said. "So I decided to forego treatment, and went on the trip."

"Gordon would just refuse to deal with things," Beverly Fogarty remembered. "I dragged him to the pulmonologist. I did a lot of research and reading."

According to the research, the infusion treatment isn't guaranteed to be 100 percent effective against the effects of Alpha-1, which often attacks the lungs and leads to emphysema, but the sooner a patient begins treatment, the greater the effectiveness.

"It was very frustrating for me, because I tend to confront problems and take care of them," Beverly said. "In Gordon's family, people never talked about their health. If they were really under the weather, they said they were okay.

"He didn't start it when he returned either," she added. "It was a long time after that."

"This sailing trip" was anything but a small excursion. Determined to accomplish a major goal on his bucket list, Gordon had signed up as a crew member on the Bark Europa, an old-fashioned 1911 tall ship. The two-month voyage would embark from Tierra del Fuego around Cape Horn through Antarctic waters, finishing in Cape Town, South Africa.

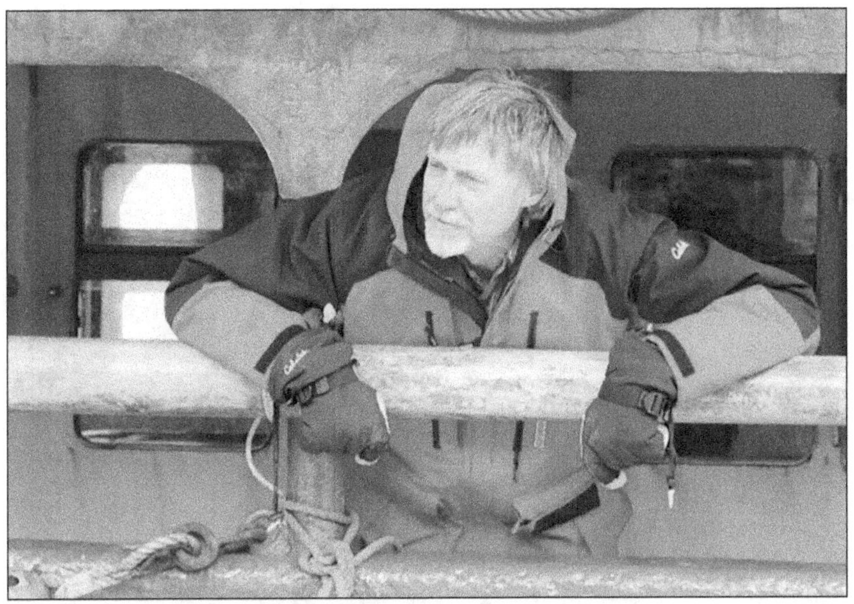

Gordon on railing looking out at sea

And, if the trifling matter of a bullet in the butt hadn't put a crimp in his Bahama sojourn twenty-seven years earlier, nothing was going to keep Gordon from this adventure. Can't breathe? So what?

"I expected the end was near and I wanted to do this," he said. "I was paid crew, meaning I paid to be there."

The voyage lasted 7,000 miles, setting sail from Ushuaia, Argentina, and voyaging around Cape Horn to the South Shetland Islands and the Antarctic Peninsula, continuing through the icebergs of the Weddell Sea toward the sub-Antarctic island of South Georgia. After a stop at Tristan da Cunha, the most remote inhabited island in the world, the final leg of the journey finished in Cape Town.

Along the way, Gordon made plenty of friends as was his custom. But he forged an especially close relationship with Andreas Kreutz, a German who planned to marry his fiancée upon arrival in Cape Town.

"During the voyage, Gordon and I shared watches, were together on lookout or at the helm, and enjoyed the beautiful scenery around

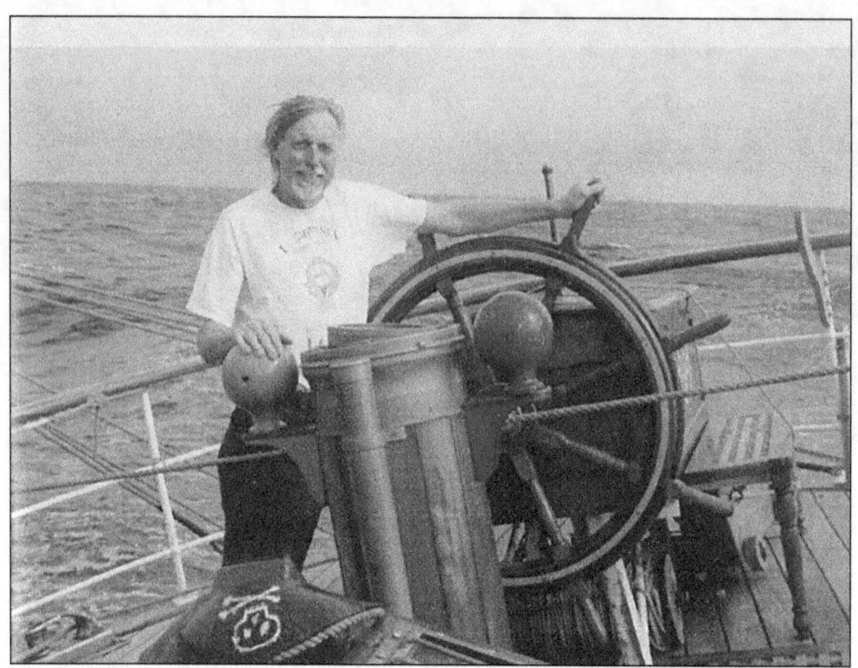

Gordon at the helm

us," Kreutz recalled. "When there was a problem with some of the machinery, I remember Gordon volunteered to help the engineer to fix it and they both did."

According to Kreutz, Gordon was really excited about getting to Tristan da Cunha, the loneliest island in the world. He had read a lot about it and knew about the famous signs posted in the main village showing distances to the island from various places worldwide. He had brought with him from home a dozen similar empty signs and a marker. To the people he befriended on board he gave each an empty sign before landing in Tristan. All crossed their fingers as they made landfall because ocean swells sometimes prevent passengers from disembarking on the island. Theirs proved to be a lucky voyage.

"I got one of the signs and wrote my hometown in Germany on it, including the distance, roughly 10,000 kilometers from Tristan," Kreutz said. "Everyone with a sign from Gordon went to the place to take pictures. Years later I received a parcel from Gordon in Germany where he sent me my sign and I still have it."

As the voyage drew closer to South Africa, Kreutz said he began to get nervous. He was meeting his fiancée, Claudia, in Cape Town and getting married for the first time. They planned to marry on an isolated beach not far from the city—just the two of them. Gordon loved their plan and was invited to join them as their only guest.

The day prior to the wedding, the couple drove over to the beach to inspect it, and found it did not live up to the photos they had seen. So they drove around and found another beach they liked much better. Unfortunately, they were unable to contact Gordon about the change in plans.

"I learned later after getting back home he had been there, but of course we hadn't," Kreutz said. "Too bad because I would have liked to have him around during the wedding ceremony."

Despite missing out on the wedding ceremony, Gordon arrived home exhilarated with another exciting adventure crossed off his bucket list.

"I felt I still had enough strength to do it, although I didn't do much rig climbing or hiking," he said. "But I always wanted to know what it would be like to be a sailor on those old-time rig ships, and it was a wonderful experience."

He also returned home with his Alpha-1 untreated and his symptoms growing worse. Upon his return, Beverly, his wife of eighteen years, delivered a bombshell. She was leaving him.

Despite their differences, the two remained close friends. Beverly agreed not to seek a divorce, so Gordon could remain on her health insurance policy.

"We got along great not living together," Beverly said. "He was always my go-to person when I needed to know how to fix things. He would drop by or give me advice over the phone."

Two years later, still struggling along without treatment, he met a new partner, Barbara, who, like Bev, took his health care into her own hands.

"You need to be treated," she said.

Barbara dragged Gordon to a pulmonologist, Dr. Terrance Barnes, who, according to Gordon, told him, "You're in a situation. It may be too late for the protein, but we've got to get you on it anyway."

Before Gordon left that day, he had an appointment to get his first infusion. Then every month, a home nurse came in to give it to him.

He noticed no difference in his condition.

"It was like nothing—very depressing," Gordon said. As the years passed, his world began to grow smaller.

"My life was very small," Gordon said. "It involved no stairs and being very careful about how far I went. I had to get people to shop for me, I had to watch how I slept, and everything depended on the parameter of being able to walk 15 feet.

"I could see my mortality reflected in the eyes of my friends," he added.

Several years after the Antarctica voyage, Andreas Kreutz was visiting an aunt in Chicago and contacted Gordon to visit him in Pentwater for a few days. The difference between the Gordon of the Europa voyage and the Gordon he saw now astounded him.

"He had told me about his disease, but I didn't know that it was so bad," Kreutz said. "When I saw him he couldn't walk five steps without resting afterwards for a minute or so.

"He took me out one day in his sailboat on the lake and we had a wonderful time," he said. "When we got back to the pier, it was terrible for him. Just the two steps up caused him to rest for the next two minutes because he didn't get enough air through his lungs."

In early 2014, Gordon again sought treatment with his pulmonologist.

"Things got really bad and I went back to Barnes," Gordon said. "He said, 'Wow, you've really slowed.' And I said, 'Is there anything we can do?'"

There was nothing short of a lung transplant.

By this point, Gordon's Alpha-1 had created emphysema and chronic obstructive pulmonary disease by destroying the alveoli, the tiny air sacs of the lungs that allow for rapid exchange of gasses. Because of this destruction and loss of surface area, more air in the lungs did not equate to more oxygen. The additional loss of elastic tissue would not allow Gordon to exhale at a normal rate.

According to Dr. Reda Girgis, medical director of Spectrum Health's lung transplant program, the first medical tests on Gordon showed his total lung capacity at 160 percent of the normal value. However, due to the obstruction and dynamic hyperinflation of his lungs, he could not exhale the air. At any given time, Gordon's lungs contained more than three times as much air as a normal pair of lungs, which explains the constant gasping he refers to.

A common measure of lung function is the forced expiratory volume-one second (FEV1), a measure of how much air can be exhaled in one second following a deep inhalation. Values of between 80 and 120 percent of the average value are considered normal. Gordon's first FEV1 produced a value of 23 percent.

There was no guarantee that Gordon would even qualify for a transplant. At 66, his age was against him. And he would have to undergo a battery of physical and psychological tests. Then, if approved, the right pair of lungs would have to be available—a large pair, because he was a big man. For all the elements to fall into place was at best a long shot. For them to fall into place before time ran out was even less likely.

It would take a miracle to bring Gordon back from the edge of the abyss.

Fortunately, within six months, that miracle would happen.

10

The Swimmer: Sinking Fast

"Athletes know when the time has come to move on."

—Fred Nelis

OR THE NEXT TWELVE YEARS, Fred's life would be one of vigilance.

He preserved his high level of fitness, continuing his rigorous training, and managed to maintain his ejection fraction in the low thirties. Fred continued his active life as father, breadwinner, and swim coach. Neither he nor Jean had the time or inclination to give in to despair and depression.

"The kids were little when Fred was diagnosed," Jean said. "We were busy and had to carry on with the normal demands of a family. I didn't have a lot of time to think about things. We decided we had hope and weren't going to dwell on the bad."

But Fred also learned to monitor himself closely for any changes in his health.

Things were going well until October 12, 2006. That was the morning Fred awoke unable to see clearly out of his right eye. He lost no time getting to his ophthalmologist. The verdict was not good. He'd suffered a stroke in that eye.

How? Why? He'd had no evidence of coronary artery blockage. Had his blood pressure dropped too low, due, perhaps, to the drugs he was taking? When blood pressure drops too low, blood flow doesn't have the pressure to get through the bone surrounding the optic nerve, thus causing stroke.

After alerting his cardiologist, Fred went to the University of Michigan Kellogg Eye Center. There he received more troubling news. Yes, he'd had a stroke, and yes, it had resulted in damage to the optic nerve. And yes, there was a 50/50 chance the same thing could happen to his other eye.

Ever the optimist, Fred preferred to bank on the lucky 50 percent chance that an episode wouldn't happen. But unfortunately, the unlucky 50 percent won out. A couple of months later, he had a stroke in his left eye.

"Until this incident, I never had anger regarding my plight," Fred said. "But this hit me hard. I was faced with an almost impossible choice: either stop my heart meds and take my chances, or go blind."

Shaken to the bone at what he felt to be his cardiologist's blasé attitude toward his plight, he decided to seek out a new doctor.

His internist, Dr. David Young, contacted Dr. Mike Dickinson in Grand Rapids. In late 2006, Fred and Jean met with Dickinson, who cheerfully assured him that of all the things he might die of, heart failure wasn't one of them. Well, that was a relief. But what about his eyes?

Dickinson prescribed a change in medication, taking Fred off the problematic beta blockers. His eyesight never returned to normal, but his eyes seemed to stabilize—either that or he adjusted and learned to compensate for his new disability.

Fast forward to March 2011. Fred's swimming was not going well, and he made a difficult decision. In order to avoid any further embarrassment while swimming in meets, he decided that the competition he entered that month would be his last.

"I saw no reason to humiliate myself in front of my friends," he said. "Athletes know when the time has come to move on."

An uncanny dread was again creeping into Fred's mind, and unlike his first experience in 1993, this time he thought he knew the cause: the final fatal stages of end-stage heart failure.

Dr. Dickinson was not so sure, however.

Uncertain about the cause, he began the search for the usual suspects. He didn't rule out heart failure, but the results of another metabolic stress test showed no change in Fred's fitness level. An echocardiogram confirmed ejection fraction at his normal 30 percent. So what was going on?

Christmas of 2012 was not a merry one. On December 26, Fred was back in the Holland Hospital ER with bronchial spasms. He was unable to catch his breath at rest. More prescriptions were added to his med cocktail: Advair and a rescue inhaler.

But nothing was working. The next step was an allergy specialist—another dead end. A metabolic stress test with a pulmonologist indicated that Fred was in the 97th percentile of performers—another dead end.

Throughout the six months of on-and-off testing, Fred continued to swim, even though it became so depressing that he found himself looking for reasons to miss practice. That was when his training partner, Dr. Steve Van Wylen, suggested that acid reflux might be the cause of his breathing problems, and put Fred on a six-week regimen of strong antacids to see if the condition improved.

It didn't. Time for an endoscopy.

The results of that procedure were definitive: they showed severe reflux. His esophagus was dangerously inflamed.

"Without a doubt, you have silent acid reflux," Van Wylen informed Fred. "If you had regular reflux, you would have been miserable."

Van Wylen scheduled his friend for a procedure called a Nissan, an operation that prevents stomach contents, especially acids, from flowing back into the esophagus. "I've done maybe 1,000 of these surgeries," the doctor told Fred and Jean. "But I must say that your esophagus rates in the top 10 for damage."

Surgery was scheduled ASAP. Meanwhile, Fred met with his dentist, Dr. Brittany Mailloux, who, during a routine checkup the previous month, had also mentioned the possibility of reflux, as enormous damage to the enamel was evident in Fred's otherwise healthy teeth. Now she dropped another bomb. "We need to pull your wisdom teeth. And then you'll need 28 crowns."

Twenty-eight crowns? That was virtually every tooth in his mouth! Faced with more surgery, extensive dental work, and ongoing heart problems, Fred wondered if he'd be waking up anytime soon from what had become a continuing nightmare.

On May 31, 2013, Fred checked into Holland Hospital for the Nissan surgery.

Everything was proceeding as planned, Fred was fully prepped for surgery, he had kissed Jean, and was rolled down the hall to the OR with about a half-dozen heart leads attached to his chest. Then, just as he heard Dr. Van Wylen say, "Lights out," things suddenly screeched to a halt.

The anesthesiologist had stopped the operation because Fred was in full atrial fibrillation.

Back Fred went to his room, to wait for clearance from Dr. Dickinson. At nearly 5:00 p.m., a cardiologist from his group gave the green light and the operation went as planned, without a hitch.

The A-fib diagnosis was another unexpected curve ball. While the condition is fairly common in the general population, it's a serious threat for patients with additionally compromised hearts. Yet unsettling as it was, the diagnosis was something of a relief. Crazy as it seemed, all the testing Fred had undergone that past year failed to detect the condition. At least he knew now why he'd been feeling so miserable for so long.

Since untreated A-fib can lead to blood clots, Fred was put on a month's regimen of the blood thinner Xarelto. On July 2, he underwent a cardioversion, an attempt to shock the heart back into proper rhythm. Then he and Jean sat back to wait for the results. His follow-up appointment with Dr. Dickinson was sobering.

"When Dr. Dickinson entered the room, I could tell by his face that the news wasn't good," Fred said. "The cardioversion didn't work; I was still in A-fib."

As far as Fred was concerned, the die was now cast. He laid out his plans to get all dental work done immediately because he knew that nothing would be permitted should he be hospitalized. He knew by this point that it wasn't if he would be going into the hospital, but when.

On August 9, Fred's wisdom teeth were taken out. One site in particular gave him constant pain. The problem turned out to be a molar; the solution was a root canal. The following week began the ordeal of the 28 crowns. This endurance test was made even more pleasant by his internist's order of no sedation. Fred had to remain awake because of his heart condition.

"I was feeling so terrible by this time that I'd stopped swimming entirely by mid-October, and was just praying we'd make it in time," he said.

On October 25, the final 8 crowns were done. But just as the last cap was being fitted, it broke. It would be another week before the replacement was ready. With 27 caps done and just one to go, Fred and Jean responded to this latest setback with their usual "laughter is the best medicine" ingenuity. Their annual Halloween party was the next day and Fred brought the house down as the Tooth Fairy, while Jean was dressed as a crown with the logo "27 + 1" on her costume.

On November 7, Fred returned to Holland Hospital for a heart catheterization. The results were sent to Spectrum Health in Grand Rapids, where Fred was scheduled for a follow-up cath. The follow-up cath concurred with the previous week's results, and Fred and Jean were asked if they'd prepared an overnight bag.

It was obvious that the cath results were cause for concern.

Fred settled in for the first of a few hundred IV pokes and was hooked up to a telemetry box with five leads attached to his chest. This was somewhat expected, but his next visitor was not: Dr. Asghar Khagani, one of the world's leading heart transplant surgeons.

"I knew who Dr. Khagani was but didn't put things together until later the following week," Fred said. "We had a short, cordial conversation; I just assumed he was making rounds and had stepped into my room."

On Friday, the "Team" entered Fred's room. Something was up—something Fred wasn't prepared for. "Don't even think about going home," the doctor told him. "On Monday, we're going to implant a pacemaker/defibrillator for your safety."

The concern on the team's faces made the gravity of his situation clear. Although he'd managed to avoid having the placement of the device for the last three years, Fred realized that time was up. It was happening.

The implant was successful and Fred was back in his room by noon on Monday. When the team visited him on afternoon rounds, they informed him he would be prepared for another procedure—a colonoscopy.

Fred did not yet realize it, but plans were afoot to get a battery of tests and exams out of the way as the clinicians prepared him for transplant consideration.

The day after the colonoscopy, while Fred and Jean were walking the halls, Dr. Dickinson approached them and asked Fred if he'd like to receive a heart pump the next day. His patient didn't need to read between any lines. Things must be pretty bad, even very bad, for Dickinson to propose a second surgery in a week.

The pump Dickinson was referring to was an LVAD. Unlike an artificial heart, the LVAD does not replace the heart. As an "assist device," its function is to help the heart do its job. This can mean the difference between life and death for someone whose heart is too weak to pump on its own, or who is waiting for a heart transplant.

The surgery went well, but the aftermath was another story. After spending a couple of days in the ICU, Fred was moved to 7 Heart, the floor where, when he finally received his transplant, he would spend most of his days.

Fred soon discovered that implanting an LVAD was a far more complicated procedure than getting a little old pacemaker.

For the foreseeable future, he would be hooked up to what he referred to as a "Batman-like utility belt." Around his waist was a heavy belt containing three pouches. Two of the compartments contained lithium batteries, while the middle section held the pump controller.

"Imagine a not-so-small hole in the abdomen, about three inches from the belly button," Fred describes it. "That's where a plastic-shrouded electrical cord entered the skin and wove its way to the tiny pump attached to the bottom of my heart."

Then there was the dressing change. Because of the wound—which, it turned out, never closed fully—a daily dressing was applied to prevent infection and offer stability for the driveline. This was not a simple procedure. It took 45 minutes, and because less than half the nurses were LVAD-trained, a family member had to be trained to perform the task when Fred went home.

About the middle of the second week, Jean was pressed into service. Soon she was as good as the trained nurses, and for the next seven months, Fred and his wife spent an intimate 45 minutes every day looking into a hole in his abdomen.

In addition to the dressing change, both needed to be trained to troubleshoot the controller and battery pack. Each battery would sound an alarm when it got low, signaling time to change out the spent unit for a fresh one. They were cautioned to remove the proper cable to avoid disconnecting the fully charged battery instead of the spent unit.

"The incision site was always uncomfortable," Fred recalled.

A five-inch opening was made just left and down from the left breast, and four to five inches of bone had been cut at the top of the sternum. Only a short portion was cut to prevent potential problems with scar tissue later when Fred would receive his transplant.

The sternum was never wired shut, and for the entire time up to the transplant—seven months later—was sore and tender. The slightest jar or bump would send Fred reeling.

Saturday, November 30, might have been just another day had it not been for the sudden commotion in Fred's room. Startled and bleary eyed, he awoke to find half of the nurses on 7 Heart crowded around him, bombarding him with anxious questions. "Are you all right?" "Do you feel funny?" "Can you talk?"

It turned out that the telemetry unit had set off an alarm, instigating a Code Blue–an indication that the patient is in cardiopulmonary arrest.

"There I was, in a state of adrenalin-induced excitement with little explanation as to what had just happened," Fred said. "Finally part of the team arrived for a look-see and concluded that a 'suction event' had occurred."

A suction event is a drop in the rate of velocity of the pump, when there isn't enough blood volume to sustain the left ventricular flow. The pump continues to pull blood out at such a rate that it creates "suction" in the ventricle. A suction event can be caused by a number of conditions, including dehydration, blood loss, medications, position changes, and other factors.

When Jean arrived, she commented on how ashen Fred looked. He was surprised; he thought he was feeling fine. But a stroll around the floor, which he usually looked forward to, proved otherwise. He began feeling strange, then terrible.

The on-call physician was again paged to Fred's room. Upon the doctor's arrival, the portable X-ray unit was called "STAT" to his room. He remembers the concern in everyone's eyes. Jean called the kids, most of whom had returned home—Lindsey to Denver, Jami to Indianapolis, and Heather to Battle Creek. Only Kelly lived in the area.

For the second time that day, it was all hands on deck as Fred's telemetry alerted staff to another event. He was immediately moved to the ICU and then to the procedure room for a chest tube. His left lung had collapsed, and time was of the essence.

When Fred returned to his room, daily blood draws were ordered. Within a couple of days, his white blood cell count began to soar, exceeding the normal range of 4,000 to 11,000 per microliter of blood to reach 50,000. He was so sick that, as he put it, "feeling terrible would have been an improvement."

X-rays showed something on the left side and also confirmed that his lung had not fully inflated. He underwent a thoracotomy, a procedure that involves cleaning the incision site of pus, dead tissue, and dried blood.

Usually a thoracotomy provides relief. In Fred's case, however, it just made him feel worse. Blood cultures revealed a tag team of infections, from E coli to yeast.

How had that happened? The cause was a tiny tear in the bowel that occurred during the LVAD implant. Massive doses of IV anti-fungal drugs and antibiotics were administered.

Fred's desire for company was at low ebb. Little food, less sleep, an onslaught of chemicals, and a clogged-up GI tract made life agony. Time was the only constant, and it seemed like the hospital had plenty to spare. What should have been about a two-week stay had turned into a month, with no end in sight. Finally, however, the long-awaited release came.

"After 36 days, some I can't even remember, I was able to depart the hospital under my own power," Fred said. "It was so nice to see the hospital in the rearview mirror, I almost cried."

Getting home was fabulous, but the new normal brought the hospital home with him. Fred had a visiting nurse three times a week. Supplies for the LVAD dressing were delivered every Monday. Each morning for three weeks, Jean started the day with an IV drip of antibiotics.

"Although I could have done without that, it was a remarkable time of quiet togetherness," Fred recalled.

Fred was isolated at home until February. Then he was put on a strict routine: cardiac rehab three times a week, with Jean by his side in case of pump controller problems.

By March, life was stabilizing. He was feeling much stronger and had gained back 15 of the 50 pounds he lost in the hospital. Twice a week he was back at the pool, unable to enter the water himself, but still coaching the US Masters Swim program. He also lifted weights and walked the malls with Jean, "to see how many steps I could put on her Fitbit."

But on March 5, he was back at Spectrum with a clot in his LVAD.

"Of all the times I was in the hospital, this visit was especially cruel," Fred said. "I'd been feeling great, had a routine going, the weather was good enough to venture outside."

What was pointed out was how serious this problem could become. A clot in the LVAD isn't the same as a clot in an artery. This tiny little pump spins at anywhere from 2,800 rpm to 3,500 rpm, and while the odds of blowing a clot into the blood stream are remote, the sludge that was forming in the pump could slow down the impeller, or worse, stop the pump altogether.

Fred was pumped full of anti-coagulants. On March 12, he was listed "1A," the highest priority for a transplant. It was a dire situation: because of his size, he needed a big man's heart. And his blood type was O-positive, the most difficult match for a heart transplant.

As usual, however, Fred had ideas of his own.

"My memory was still very fresh from a 36-day stay that included misery, pain, dread, and time lost," Fred said. "My thoughts were raging."

Prior to his transplant listing on March 12, Fred felt the case needed to be made that the LVAD might help reduce heart stress and permit healing or improvement. He held out hope that his heart function could improve with the aid of the assist device, just as it had in 1994 with his insistence on swimming.

Fred also had grave concerns that his body would reject any transplanted organ as a foreign body. After all, hadn't it been a virus that was most likely the culprit of all of his heart problems in the first place?

Another concern was that, despite his grave illness, he did not perceive an imminent threat to his life. He worried that there might be another person out there with a more critical need.

Finally, Fred felt a keen moral dilemma that another person had to die for him to have the potential to receive the gift of life. This awareness and reverence for the dual nature of the transplant process is something that remained strong in Fred throughout his transplant process and remains strong today. At times, he agonizes that another died so that he might live.

"Every day someone from the transplant clinic came in for a pep talk to get my permission for listing," Fred recalled. "It was a time for real soul searching, and I was just not ready to make a decision.

I think the staff got tired of my stubbornness and began to work on Jean," he added. "It took them a week, but eventually everyone wore me down."

He left Spectrum Health on March 16, 2014, to anxiously, and somewhat reluctantly, await "the call."

11

The Call:
The Transplant Team's Perspective

"Some people cheer, others cry, others go silent,
others hang up in shock."

—Krista Veine,
Spectrum Health Transplant Program Manager

T HE RAMIFICATIONS and implications of organ transplant for both the donor family and the recipient are lifelong ones. Relationships can be forged with strangers who become extended family. And even if the two sides of the equation are never brought together, this unique process gives birth to an entire inner life of philosophical and spiritual challenges and curious pondering of what-ifs.

Operating at the fulcrum of that delicate balance is a team of professionals—nurses, technicians, transplant coordinators, cardiologists, pulmonologists, surgeons, and others—who must constantly live with these highest of stakes. Their challenge is to provide the expertise, care, and compassion necessary to see people through some of the most physically and emotionally demanding days of their lives without being overwhelmed by the enormous waves of emotion that continuously flow through the transplant setting.

In addition to these challenges, the professional demands of such a long and complicated process of diagnosis, testing, evaluation, listing, transplant, recovery, and rehabilitation are also great. The process of being listed for transplant for both the prospective patient and his or her caregivers is a whirlwind of action and then an extended wait, not unlike characterizations of the armed forces during wartime.

In 1984, Congress passed the National Organ Transplant Act, which established the Organ Procurement and Transplantation Network (OPTN) to ensure fair and equitable allocation of donated organs. It also provided grants for the establishment of organ procurement organizations, such as Gift of Life Michigan and equivalent groups in other states. Two years later, the US Department of Health and Human Services awarded the national OPTN contract to the United Network for Organ Sharing (UNOS). UNOS established the current organ sharing system, collects and publishes data pertaining to transplants, and works to increase the number of organs available for transplantation.

Transplant centers such as Spectrum Health are in constant contact with UNOS and their state organ procurement organization, seeking a match when donated organs become available. But how exactly does a patient proceed from a diagnosis of heart or lung failure to awaking with a new organ and a new lease on life?

We have already seen some of the steps that must be taken when Fred was initially listed for transplant at Henry Ford Hospital, and when he was finally convinced to become listed at Spectrum Health. The full process is even more complex and emotionally fraught.

Typically, as in the case of Fred and Dr. Dickinson, an advanced heart or lung failure patient will have an established relationship with a cardiologist or pulmonologist, who orders a transplant evaluation to be completed within a two-week period.

Once a prospective recipient is accepted, the patient is assigned a transplant coordinator, who initiates a round of testing that includes more than twenty items. The patient and his or her coordinator meet with a battery of specialists, including infectious disease specialists, radiologists, phlebotomists, psychologists, pharmacists, dietitians, and of course, the surgical team.

There is much to consider, including the patient's age, state of mind, attitude toward physical therapy, and potential compliance with their daily regimen of immunosuppressant drugs. Finally, the team also weighs factors such as family support and other, not-so-easily quantifiable psychological factors, such as determination, persistence, and will to live.

"It's not only our job to evaluate but also help the patient to overcome any barriers," said Spectrum Health Transplant Program Manager Krista Veine.

Barriers to transplant take many forms, some financial, some dietary, and some having to do with risk factors such as smoking and other detrimental behaviors. The job of the transplant team, and most especially the coordinator, is to help the patient overcome those barriers by connecting them to resources such as financial experts, nutritionists, social workers, and psychologists.

"Sometimes we are successful and sometimes we are not," Veine said. "If we are, the next step is for the patient to be placed on the organ wait list."

GORDON VELDMAN HAD a number of such barriers. The most obvious being his age, but there were others that did not make his case a slam dunk for approval.

A Spectrum Health team of psychologists published a study in the peer-reviewed *Journal of Clinical Psychology in Medical Settings* in 2015. The study detailed the pre-transplant biomedical and psychological evaluations of an anonymous, prospective double lung transplant candidate referred to by the pseudonym "Mr. Jeffrey Phillips." Under federal law, the identity of such subjects is strictly confidential. Gordon, however, was proud to share with Fred and many others that he was (quite obviously) the subject of the paper.

Mr. Phillips' caregiver plan was difficult to finalize because he was estranged from his family-of-origin due to religious disagreements. Despite strong medical recommendations, he had not been using portable bottled oxygen when he left his house. He denied depression symptoms but reported 'astronomical' feelings of anxiety, and he offered several peculiar statements (e.g., 'Logic is my supreme commander.'). In regards to substance abuse, he reported a distant history of cigarette smoking, no alcohol abuse, and no drug use. However, a urine toxicology screen...demonstrated recent cannabis use... Mr. Phillips was judged to be a high risk for lung transplantation due to lack of an organized post-surgical caregiver plan, inconsistent use of portable oxygen, self-reported high anxiety, recent cannabis use, deception about cannabis use, and peculiar statements.

"Mr. Phillips" was given a score of 38 on the Stanford Integrated Psychosocial Assessment for Transplant (SIPAT), which falls into the "minimally acceptable" transplant candidate range.

The following month, when "Mr. Phillips" was re-evaluated, he "offered fewer anxious and peculiar statements, and his romantic partner (Barbara) agreed to be his post-surgical caregiver." His SIPAT score was recalculated to 17, putting him into the "good" candidate range.

WAITING FOR THE CALL

The next phase can often be one of the most challenging for patients, according to transplant team members. Many advanced heart failure patients, like Fred, come to the wait list on LVAD support. These devices are keeping them alive to bridge them to transplant. The only treatment for their disease is a transplanted organ.

"They are waiting to live," said Becky Shore, Spectrum Health Transplant Program Manager. "Essentially they are dying, and part of our job is to encourage them and to make sure their testing is up to date until the call comes in."

When an organ becomes available, the transplant coordinator is the first to evaluate a possible match. There is standard work in determining basic exclusion criteria, including, though not limited to, size, weight, donor and organ quality, travel distance, and blood type.

Size is a factor that is often not the first thing the public thinks of in terms of the transplant process, but it is a very decisive factor. A large man's heart and lungs will simply not fit in the chest cavity of a smaller man or most women, not to mention, a child in need of a transplant. As large men, Fred and Gordon both needed large donor organs from a larger-than-average donor.

"I liked to joke that if one of the mountain gorillas ever went missing from the Detroit Zoo, we would know the reason," Fred said.

THE CALL

Following the standard workup, the transplant coordinator will make a recommendation to the surgeon, who decides whether or not to undertake the transplant. When the surgeon decides the organ is a match, it is the coordinator's job to call the patient in to prep for surgery.

Both Veine and Shore concur that when that call successfully goes through, the response can provide the emotional and professional motivation that keeps a transplant staff going through the hard times.

"Some people cheer, others cry, others go silent, others hang up in shock," said Veine.

"Honestly, calling the patient to say we have found a possible match is probably the most rewarding part of the job," said Shore. "Often they are speechless. They may be overcome with sadness for the donor and donor family, but filled with joy that they will be given the chance to live.

"Most are happy and excited," Shore added. "It is their last option. There is no other option. If you say no today, you don't know if there will be another option."

THE ARRIVAL

Another moment in the process, fraught with its own excitement, professional dedication, fear, and hope, is the arrival of the donated organ at the destination hospital where the recipient lies in the OR prepped for what is hoped to be the final lifesaving surgery of his or her life.

The organ may have been recovered at the same hospital or at one in a nearby city. Quite often, however, the organ recovery team (usually one or more surgeons, a coordinator, and other technical staff) is forced to travel to a distant city or even to fly to another state, and time is of the essence. Under the standard practice of preserving the organ on ice, the team has a mere six hours or so of travel time after removal until a heart or lung becomes ischemic, or damaged and unusable due to a lack of blood flow.

When the organ arrives, in the care of the organ recovery team, it is often accompanied by sirens and the squealing of tires pulling up to the emergency room entrance, in the interest of making every second count. The patient is usually already under anesthesia, although the nervous family members are awake at the window, waiting and watching and praying for the organ to arrive safely.

The recovery team rushes the organ to the OR, where it undergoes tests to confirm its viability. Sometimes the recovery team is tasked with the double duty of carrying out or assisting in the transplant. Usually, however, a different surgical team awaits the arrival and handoff of the organ.

THE OTHER SIDE OF THE EQUATION

The transplant equation is perhaps best summed up in the sign that Fred hung on the door of his recovery room on 7 Heart during his recovery from surgery: "Only the Father knows the balance between grief and gratitude."

In the case of organ donation from a deceased donor, for every moment of joy, there is a corresponding one of sorrow. For every patient with a new lease on life, there is a family that must move on from the tragic consequences of the loss of a loved one. That situation is approached with the utmost care, respect, and reverence for the life that is lost and the one that may continue.

Gift of Life Michigan and other state and regional organ and tissue recovery agencies spell out their process, under federal law, with a clear set of guidelines and mandates. The last item in these guidelines states:

After a moment of silence in honor of the donor, surgery begins. Organs are removed, cooled, and preserved with special solutions. Surgical teams immediately return to their respective transplant hospitals with the organs to perform the transplant surgeries.

This last bullet point is important and can't be stressed enough. The process of organ recovery is carried out with the utmost respect and reverence for the donor and donor's family.

"Remember," said Steve Ashley, an organ recovery coordinator at an Indiana hospital in an inside look at the organ recovery process provided by the *Indy Star*. "This room becomes sacred when a family entrusts us with one of their most precious possessions."

He read a few words about the woman no one in the room knew, but who was the reason they were there that night. He shared personal messages from her family, including a few inside jokes, and then pulled a laminated card from his pocket.

The middle-aged woman on the operating table, he reminded everyone, was both dear to her husband, children and other family members, and a hero. To honor her, he said, everyone in the room should conduct themselves as 'though the family were present.'

Then, there was a moment of silence, heads bowed, eyes down. Most surgeries do not egin with such a preface. But this was no routine surgery. Although the woman on the operating table continued to breathe with the help of a ventilator, she had been declared dead a day earlier.

WALK OF HONOR

NOTE FOR THE READER: Prior to the surgical procedure, many hospitals pay final respects and honor to the donor and family with the staff and friends silently lining the corridor/halls. It's very hard to do justice in words to this moving and emotional act, but numerous online videos can be found by Googling "Walk of Honor."

12

Fred vs. Fred

*"Only the Father knows the balance
between grief and gratitude."*

—FRED NELIS

REBECCA MARIE VOGELSANG, "Becca" to her friends and family, was a busy and popular senior at Forest Hills Eastern High School, a sparkling, brand-new facility located in the prosperous Grand Rapids suburb of Ada. On the morning of Saturday, March 1, 2008, the 17-year-old was on her way to a choreography meeting and rehearsal for the school musical. That year's production was *Copacabana*, and she had a leading role.

Although she was tired and had homework to finish for the upcoming week, she also had a lot of things to be excited about. The musical promised to be a success, and Becca had just been accepted to the University of Michigan where she planned to study molecular biology.

Becca was gratified, though not completely surprised, to be accepted. After all, she had invested a great deal of time and effort in her studies. She was a member of the National Honor Society, had won a varsity athletic letter as a member of the bowling team, and overall was a bright and active teen with myriad interests and extracurricular activities. In the fall, she would be off to Ann Arbor, where she would join her older sister, Amanda, a sophomore studying business.

If UM seemed a natural fit, her choice of major was a more difficult decision. Becca loved singing and dancing, starting lessons at age three with the Ada Dance Academy Performing Company and progressing to the Blue Lake International Ensemble and annual performances with the Moscow Ballet. She performed in France, Germany, and Denmark, and took master classes in New York and Chicago.

Becca also loved languages and linguistics. She especially enjoyed studying Spanish, Japanese, and Chinese and looked forward to traveling to these countries to immerse herself in the language and culture.

In the end though, it was her desire to help others that determined her decision. She wanted to improve and save lives by finding new treatments and cures for devastating illnesses, and she felt confident and satisfied in her choice of molecular biology. Her mother was chief investment officer at Van Andel Institute, a Grand Rapids-based biomedical research institute, and she saw firsthand the difference molecular research could make, leading to clinical trials for cancer, Parkinson's, and other diseases.

The desire to help others prompted Becca's devotion to teaching Sunday school at St. Robert of Newminster Church and volunteering at God's Kitchen, a Catholic Services food and pantry program. She was a loving girl, unembarrassed to show affection with hugs or to lie on the sofa with her head in her mother's lap. It was during one of those moments of bonding that she told her mother, right after receiving her first driver's license, that she planned to sign an organ donor card as soon as she was old enough.

It was a cold March that year and the two-lane county roads between her house and the high school were filled with icy patches where the snow thawed and refroze, making driving a challenge. When the choreography meeting started and Becca still hadn't arrived, her friends and cast mates became worried. It wasn't like her to arrive late without calling. When they called her home to check on her, her parents, Phillip and Kathleen Vogelsang, began to worry.

They soon discovered the cause of Becca's delay when they received a phone call from the Spectrum Health Emergency Department. Becca had hit a patch of ice near a busy intersection with her Toyota Camry, forcing her into a side-impact collision with an oncoming pickup truck. She had been taken to the intensive care unit at Spectrum Health Butterworth Hospital with severe head injuries and placed on life support.

Word quickly spread, and classmates and friends gathered to pray Sunday afternoon at the family's home church. Monday was quickly organized as "Blue for a Better Becca Day" at school, and students dressed in blue clothes to show their support. During the school day, students autographed banners and made get-well posters, delivering them to the hospital that night and visiting over the next several days.

Becca couldn't have visitors in the ICU, but her father, Phil, took time to meet with students and friends who gathered in the hospital waiting room, sharing memories with many and playing cards with those who lingered, unwilling to go home just yet.

Phil and Kathy never spoke to their bright, lively, talented daughter again.

For five days she lay in a coma with brain damage. As her brain tissue began to deteriorate and monitors showed no signs of brain activity, Phil and Kathy made the difficult decision to take their daughter off life support. Becca passed away on the evening of Thursday, March 6.

The five days in the ICU waiting room, and those that followed, were a necessary blur. Kathy remembers being comforted by a priest at the hospital, and also recalls being approached by a representative of Gift of Life Michigan to discuss the possibility of organ donation.

The non-profit Gift of Life Michigan is the state's only federally designated organ and tissue recovery program, providing all services necessary for organ donation to occur in Michigan. The organization serves as a liaison between donors, hospitals, and transplant centers and maintains the Michigan Organ Donor Registry in partnership with the Michigan Secretary of State.

At first, the idea of removing her daughter's organs to implant them in someone else was shocking and unthinkable. It was not something a grieving parent should ever have to consider. After making the gut-wrenching decision to remove their beautiful daughter from life support, how could they be faced with another such agonizing decision? After talking with Phil, however, Kathy remembered her conversation with Becca from the previous year, and the couple did not hesitate to sign the necessary paperwork.

Becca's funeral and memorial service packed the 800-seat St. Robert of Newminster Church to standing room capacity. Rev. Msgr. R. Louis Stasker, the pastor to the parish of 2,600 families, had the unenviable task of providing solace and trying to make some semblance of sense out of a tragedy that affected hundreds of people. Kathy and Phil were told he did a remarkable job of providing comfort, although they have little recollection of the words he spoke.

Kathy said that she and Phil didn't know what they would do for the first year, but they did not have the option of falling apart and succumbing completely to grief. They still had two other daughters to raise—Amanda, who had to return alone to finish her sophomore year of college, and Laura, 13, a seventh-grader who would soon follow in her older sisters' footsteps at Forest Hills Eastern.

For Laura, it was a very difficult first year.

"Laura took on some of Rebecca's traits, which, I found out, is pretty normal," Kathy recalled. "She would watch the same TV shows that Rebecca used to watch and wear her T-shirts. Rebecca was very affectionate, and Laura became like that, putting her head in my lap and so on."

Despite these coping mechanisms, Kathy said there was a lot of anger underlying that first year of grieving for the adolescent Laura.

"Laura refused to talk to grief counselors and would not talk to adults at our church," Kathy said. "She had a meltdown after a year."

It was early in that first year that the family received a letter from Michigan Gift of Life, which for Kathy and Phil, provided a turning point in their grieving process. The letter thanked the couple for their generosity and specifically detailed the ways that Becca's organs had provided a final chance at life for seven seriously ill patients.

It was a letter that might seem alarming at first, but in the end provided enormous comfort. Because of Becca and the Vogelsangs' generosity, seven people with end-stage organ failure now had a new chance at life. Their young daughter's gift of life had provided new hope for seven people in desperate need of a heart, liver, pancreas, two kidneys, and two lungs.

Other letters followed.

"We received a letter from a young mother with two little girls who sent a photo," Kathy said.

That young mother was the grateful recipient of Becca's lungs.

"The picture helped," Kathy said. "It really is cathartic in the grieving process to know people are living because of your loved one's generosity. It's like they are still living," she said. "Her heart is beating in someone else's chest."

The family also received a letter from a young man who had received a kidney.

By law, the only information that Gift of Life is initially authorized to release to donor families is the patient's diagnosis, age, and sex.

After a successful transplant surgery, however, most patients feel such a profound sense of gratitude that they write the donor family a letter of thanks, which is delivered via Gift of Life as an intermediary. This letter is sometimes accompanied by photos, videos, mementos, and other personal items.

If both donor and recipient consent, personal contact information can be exchanged after one year in most, but not all, cases. In a number of instances, donor families and recipients have arranged emotional, public meetings attended by the press or smaller ones carried out in private settings. In other cases, however, grateful recipients write letter after letter, never hearing back from donor families, often giving up in disappointed frustration.

Kathy Vogelsang has a message for organ recipients who reach out to donor families, only to find disappointment that their overtures are not reciprocated.

"Everybody is on a different timeline," Kathy said. "Keep reaching out because one day we will be ready."

Through her subsequent work with donor families as a board member of Gift of Life Michigan and volunteer efforts at the Transplant Games of America, Kathy has had the opportunity to speak with many donor families and recipients.

She said that many organ recipients who reached out to donor families with words of thanks told her they were hurt and disappointed when they did not hear back from them. Kathy reassures them that grieving families are not being rude, it's just that many are not yet ready to come face-to-face with the flesh and blood reality—the living, breathing embodiment of their departed loved one.

"It's not that we don't want to hear from them or that we regret what we did," Kathy explained. "For many donor families, it may simply be too raw for them, depending on where they are in the grieving process."

In fact, nearly ten years after receiving the letters from Becca's heart and kidney recipients, she and Phil still have not contacted them.

"They probably thought I didn't want to hear from them," she says wistfully. "That's not it at all...one day we will contact them through Gift of Life."

FRED HAS MADE repeated attempts through Gift of Life to contact his donor family, but as of yet, has not heard from them. He hides his disappointment behind that ever-present smile, but it is clear that this is a circle he would desperately like to close.

Ask Fred what he'd like to say to the donor's family if given the chance, and at first he demurs.

"There are just no words to express your gratitude to a family that parted with their loved one," he said.

But he allows the idea to sprout, for just a moment, into possibility, and a beatific smile crosses his face. He is slow to speak, but it is clear he has given the matter much thought. His words seem almost to take the form of a Zen Buddhist koan:

"I'd just say: Come here…I want to give you a hug. I want you to feel my chest moving as a result of the heart that is in there. Put your ear to my rib cage. Put your hand to my pulse. Feel your loved one's pulse. Take as long as you want."

13

The Swimmer:
One Last Adventure

"Fred is the leader of the pack…Fred's mission is, 'You are going to have fun, and I'm going to make sure of it.'"

—Paula Bates

AFTER BEING DISCHARGED from the hospital in March to wait for a call that might take months, Jean knew that the best medicine for Fred would be to relax. Otherwise, she would likely find him showing up at Yost Vises. Fred and Jean's idea of fun and relaxation, however, perhaps differs from that of many people.

It includes tearing through the woods at breakneck speeds, dodging stumps and boulders on a screaming four-wheeled machine. After a ride, to relax even more, Fred might offer old friends and new acquaintances a listen at his now non-existent heartbeat, and perhaps follow that by whipping up a concoction for them known as a Duck Fart, equal parts Irish cream, Kahlua, and Crown Royal downed in a single gulp.

By now, we know a few things about Fred. He is driven by faith, duty, competition, and hard work—all sprinkled with a dash of humor and good spirits. The loves of his life are Jean, his four girls, and his grandchildren. Swimming is his passion, for which his guiding principles are the Four F's of Fun, Friends, Food, and Fitness.

But riding four-wheeled ATVs on the state forest hills and trails near the Black Mountain Lodge in Cheboygan, Michigan, is Fred's way of letting loose, communing with nature, indulging his whims, and cementing the bonds of friendship with his posse, partners in crime, kindred spirits, call them what you will, though they have a name—the Dirty Dudes and Dusty Dames.

Riding quads started as a hobby for Fred and Jean's girls, something for them to do on their grandparents' large rural acreage. But little by little, Fred and Jean picked up the bug. He bought 60-cc and 125-cc machines early on. Then, in 2001, they bought two 250-cc machines and the quads kept getting larger and more powerful, capable of climbing steep, rocky hills and attaining speeds of 70–80 mph. Then they had to buy a trailer and so on. They now own eight of the vehicles.

The Black Mountain Lodge is Fred's summer palace. If he is the restless king, the Dirty Dudes and Dusty Dames are his entourage and members of his court.

"Fred is the leader of the pack," said Paula Bates, who owns Black Mountain Lodge along with her husband, Ross. "He keeps the pack moving. Fred's mission is, 'You are going to have fun, and I'm going to make sure of it.'"

Quadding is something that Fred anticipates and thinks about during long hot days in his factory and warehouse. The excitement of feeling the rush of the wind through his hair is a pleasure he shares in common with Gordon. The spray of the mud, the donning of the gear, the fueling of the machines, climbing rugged mountains with his friends—all of these other rituals are his own.

"The anticipation and the recounting of the adventures ... that's just as good as the actual doing," Fred says. "I anticipate characters and pair up a vehicle with them."

The Dudes and Dames are serious about their riding, and the weekend-long event is fairly structured. They ride when they first arrive, despite the more than four-hour drive from Holland. Heading out to the Bluffs, they ride until it begins to get late. When they get back, they cook out on the grill and have cocktails around a giant bonfire.

"We come back, we shoot the bull, we drink, we tell stories," Fred muses. "There is comfort in the rituals."

On Saturday evening, the group heads into Cheboygan for Mass, whether they are Catholic or not, and most of them are not. Afterward they might hit one of the nicer restaurants in town like Pier 33 or the Boathouse, the two white tablecloth establishments, or the Cheboygan Brewing Company, from which Jean carries her own growler.

The Dudes and Dames is a fairly fluid group depending on the weekend, but there is a core made up of some of Fred and Jean's oldest friends.

Fred asked his old friend Kathryn Olney and her husband Bill to join the quadding adventure numerous times. She always had an excuse, but he never stopped asking. Many friends have remarked on Fred's friendly powers of persuasion, which, while persistent, fall short of annoying, and are one of his charms as a friend.

"Fred doesn't give up on you," Kathryn said. "He keeps asking. He is intent on creating a social life for everybody.

"I finally said to Bill, 'If we go one time, maybe he will stop asking,'" she recalled.

One time was all it took for her to get hooked.

"I love downhill skiing, and this is the only other thing that gives me the same rush as skiing," she said.

One of the original members of the group and the man who coined the phrase "Dirty Dudes and Dusty Dames," and designed the club's insignia, is Steve Kitsch, a Gerber Products performance manager, who along with wife, Jill, attends more than 80 percent of the weekend outings.

"When Fred gets an interest in something, he really dives into it," Kitsch shared. "He took a real liking to Black Mountain Lodge and wanted to patronize the place, so we stopped going to our other riding destinations."

Kitsch finds common ground with Fred in his own close call with mortality. In 2007, at 48, he was diagnosed with leukemia. After undergoing months of chemotherapy, Kitsch said he was at a point where he accepted the possibility of his imminent death.

"I could talk to Fred at that level, because he has been in that situation where you don't know if you are going to survive," Kitsch said.

Another point in common for the two men is a reluctance to give in to despair, despite facing long odds of survival. Kitsch says that the two things that stand out most about Fred are his generosity and a relentless drive to stay positive.

"No matter how ill and tired he looks, Fred still looks for the positive and for ways to enjoy himself with others," Kitsch said. "You knew he was in pain. You could see it, but it would never stop him. He would always say, 'Let's forge ahead.'"

Ross and Paula Bates bought Black Mountain Lodge in 2008.

Paula is a former first responder, who now works three days a week as a hygienist for a dentist in Cheboygan. Ross is a licensed mechanical contractor. His company, Global Green Mechanical Service, based in Dearborn Heights, handles the Marriott Renaissance Center, the famous "Ren Cen," in downtown Detroit. He commutes and spends four to five days per week three hours downstate in Detroit.

For a number of years, they employed a chef and were named the top restaurant in the area. The restaurant was a white tablecloth, fine dining affair, and they hired bands to play in the bar on the weekend.

The bar at the Black Mountain Lodge is a marvel of craftsmanship. It features hand carved counters and stools, and an assortment of mounted beasts—bear, elk, deer, pheasant, mallard, antelope, and a large hairy spider that drops down with the pull of a secret lever.

Given the rural location, however, there just isn't a large enough customer base. The restaurant has been closed since 2015, except for the occasional wedding or other catered gig. The place is currently up for sale.

The staffing of the entire property is now up to Ross, Paula and Wally Kew, their manager. Nonetheless, Fred and Jean's group is always welcome.

"Fred and his group have the run of the place," said Paula. "You couldn't ask for a better group of people."

"They love their four-wheeling, and they know how to have fun," adds Ross. "Fred tries to squeeze in as much life as possible."

If Fred is king of the summer palace and Bill Olney is his prime minister of fun, then Wally is a combination court jester and all-around jack of all trades. He keeps things running, knows everyone, and can get you whatever you need.

"Getting to know Fred, the rapport was instantaneous," said Wally. "The group was so nice. They embody the idea of 'always treat people the way you want to be treated.'

"They have become like family to me," he adds. "Paula told me that Fred and Jean offered to pay for my tooth implant. I would never take them up on it, but it is very generous that they would offer."

So, when Fred and the gang showed up on June 14, 2014, Fred sporting his "Batman utility belt" (LVAD), four days before his unbeknownst date with destiny, Wally and Paula were surprised to see him looking so frail.

"Paula and I were devastated," said Wally. "You could see his weight loss. He had a very gaunt look."

Fred's LVAD has two sets of batteries. One alarm tells you there is a dead battery; the backup works as a failsafe. Fred would disconnect one line as a joke. Paula did not find it amusing.

"The LVAD freaked Paula out, with the siren going off," Wally said. "Paula was livid. She thought he was gone."

Nonetheless, says Paula, "It was the same old Fred. He looked sickly before his transplant, but he was always positive, always fun and friendly—but always positive. The group helped that."

"The family seems to look at it like 'play the cards you are dealt,'" adds Ross.

And that they would do—in four short days, unbeknownst to them at the time.

It is a cool August night at Black Mountain Lodge several years later. Much has happened that will be explained in subsequent chapters. Fred and Jean have recently returned from a trip to Europe.

Kathryn Olney is nursing a rib injury she sustained earlier in the day when she flipped the quad she was riding. She is in obvious discomfort as we nurse our drinks by the campfire.

Quadding is not without risks on the steep and rocky, tree-lined, ridge-filled trails, where Fred and his friends routinely rip along at 30–40 miles per hour. Kathryn previously broke her wrist and Jean also has tipped a quad.

The fire burns brightly, night closes in, coyotes howl in the distance. Maybe we are all tired, or a bit tipsy or both. Wally cracks everyone up for some reason with his matter-of-fact storytelling.

"There was another guy who hit a deadfall and flipped his quad," says Wally. "He ended up with breast cancer. His name was Chris and his wife's name was Chris."

This breaks us all up for some reason.

Pausing to find the absurdity in another's misfortune. Taking our mind, momentarily, off our own.

REACH

Stop Trying to Live,
Start Living to Try

14

A Heartbeat's Resounding Echoes

"It was because someone took that risk that he (Richard DeVos) got that heart, and he, in keeping with his nature, wanted to give that same gift to as many people as possible. In a way that only he could do, he allowed us to start this program. I want to see that opportunity extended to as many people as possible whether that extension of life is through mechanical support or transplant of heart and lungs."

—THEODORE BOEVE, MD, Richard DeVos Endowed Director,
Spectrum Health Richard DeVos Heart and Lung
Transplant Program

TWO INDIVIDUALS would play especially key roles in the creation of a transplant center within driving distance of Fred and Gordon's remote locations in Holland and Pentwater: Richard DeVos, the billionaire co-founder of Amway Corporation, and Dr. Asghar Khaghani, the program's founding surgical director.

As a businessman, Fred has great respect and admiration for Richard DeVos; as a heart transplant patient, he has tremendous gratitude for the talents of Dr. Khaghani—the man who carried out his transplant.

"Mr. DeVos combines the tough and relentless mindset of the entrepreneur with the attitude of gratitude of a transplant patient," Fred points out. "He didn't just build the ship, he got the captain, the sailors, and the sails, and he kept pushing until that ship would sail."

"Building the ship," however, was a process that would take place over several decades. By the 1970s, downtown Grand Rapids had been dying for nearly a quarter century and was in its final throes. Warehouses and factories sat vacant, and anchor businesses, historic landmarks of the city's furniture capital heyday, were closed or on the verge of closing.

Beginning in the 1980s, however, the city began raising billions in philanthropic and public-private funding. Investments yielded a new downtown convention center, the new home of the Grand Rapids Public Museum, and the Van Andel Arena and surrounding Arena District. But the crown jewel of the city is the research and medical infrastructure investment along the Michigan Street corridor that has become known as the Medical Mile.

In 2010, officials dedicated the opening of the headquarters for the Michigan State University College of Human Medicine. The privately funded seven-story building is a 180,000-square-foot, state-of-the-art medical education facility. Jay and Betty Van Andel's billion-dollar endowment of Van Andel Institute was the gift that started the Medical Mile rolling. But it was a series of gifts and strategic development in another part of downtown that really ushered in this new era and laid the foundation for what followed.

Amway co-founder and former CEO Richard DeVos writes in his memoir *Simply Rich* about how "a community benefits from a sense of ownership by its citizens" and about "the benefits of being life enrichers" (page 222).

DeVos also credits two men in particular, Lyman Parks, the city's first African American mayor, and Dick Gillett, a prominent Grand Rapids banker, with instilling this sense of ownership and life enrichment in him and his fellow citizens, of jumpstarting the movement to bring the city back from the brink and of planting within him the seeds of philanthropy.

As downtown Grand Rapids began to come back to life during the 1980s and '90s, DeVos turned his attention to what he characterizes as his proudest accomplishment, engineering what would eventually emerge as the largest employer in the region—Spectrum Health.

But first, he had to face the greatest challenge of his life.

After years of heart issues, in 1996, his longtime Grand Rapids-based cardiologist Dr. Rick McNamara and cardiothoracic surgeon Dr. Luis Tomatis sat him down and informed him that, to continue to live, he would need a heart transplant.

Unbeknownst to DeVos, Tomatis had called every transplant center in the US to see if one would list him for a heart. They all turned him down. DeVos had many strikes against him: his age, 71 at the time, the stroke and heart attack he had suffered, diabetes, and finally, a rare AB positive blood type, which made him an extremely difficult match for a donor.

One transplant surgeon would consider the risky procedure on the condition that DeVos fly out to meet him. His name: Professor Sir Magdi Yacoub of Harefield Hospital, located in the London borough of Hillingdon.

Harefield is part of the Royal Brompton and Harefield NHS Foundation Trust, the largest heart and lung center in the United Kingdom and among the largest in Europe. Under Yacoub's leadership, the Harefield transplant program began in 1980, and by the end of the decade he and his team had performed one thousand transplants, while the hospital had become the leading UK transplant center.

DeVos was told that he would be placed last on the priority list for available hearts, behind every other UK and European Union citizen matching his blood type. He needed to stay close at hand at Harefield to undergo regular tests. The wait might be a day, or it might be months. Everything depended, as always, on the availability of a donor heart.

It took five months for DeVos to receive the call. When it came, he discovered from his cardiologist that a woman sharing his same rare blood type had come to the hospital for a lung transplant. Moreover, her failing lungs had forced her heart to compensate, which resulted in a heart with a very strong right side—just the match that his surgeons were waiting for.

Because transplanted lungs often do much better when they remain with the original donor's heart, DeVos and the woman would take part in a procedure that had come to be known as a "domino" transplant. DeVos writes of his wife, Helen, hearing the whirling blades of the chopper that would bring a new heart and lungs for the woman, who, in turn would provide her heart for DeVos.

Much in the same way that Fred and Gordon reunited in the hallways of the Meijer Heart Center, DeVos happened upon his donor while walking the halls of Harefield.

"Did you get your heart last Tuesday?" she asked.

"Yes, I did."

"You have *my* heart," she replied (DeVos, 257–58).

They stayed in touch for ten years before the woman died of cancer.

Twenty years later, DeVos' donor heart is still ticking, and its beat has gone on to have resounding effects on a community, on more than 200 West Michigan transplant patients and on the lives of those patients, their families, and loved ones, including Fred and Gordon.

After his major heart attack in 1992, but prior to his 1997 transplant, DeVos had turned his attention to what he characterizes as his proudest accomplishment, engineering the union that would eventually emerge as Spectrum Health.

Dr. Yacoub would serve as a consultant in the launch of Spectrum's transplant program, and his partner, Dr. Asghar Khaghani, would play a pivotal role in that program's success by becoming its first surgical director.

THE DEVELOPMENT OF A MASTER

Dr. Marcus Haw was appointed as a surgeon at Harefield in 1994. Today he is recognized as a world leader in pediatric congenital heart surgery.

Haw worked closely with Sir Magdi and Dr. Khaghani as Harefield became an internationally renowned center of heart and lung transplant and a leading innovator in the development of VAD surgery.

In England, after first beginning with neurosurgery, Khaghani completed his training in thoracic surgery. He decided to learn cardiac surgery as well to improve his job prospects. In 1981, Khaghani began training at Harefield with mentor professor Sir Magdi Yacoub. When he started at Harefield, Yacoub was already known internationally, although the transplant program had only recently begun.

In all, Khaghani performed more than 1,000 heart transplants and 5,000 cardiac surgeries at Harefield—he does not keep exact count. It's doubtful other surgeons will have the opportunity to perform that many. Now that there are more transplant centers and qualified surgeons, ten per year is considered a sizeable number for a surgeon, he says.

Those years of training, his work ethic, and his demeanor would catch the attention and later the heartfelt gratitude of the DeVos family. This would make him the perfect fit to help get the Richard DeVos Heart and Lung Transplant Program off the ground.

LAUNCHING A BRAND-NEW TRANSPLANT PROGRAM

After Spectrum Health received the state's third Certificate of Need authorization in January of 2010, the clock began ticking. Spectrum Health had two years to begin performing the first heart transplants in West Michigan. To maintain authorization, the program would have to perform at least twelve transplants in its second year of operation.

The race was on to build the infrastructure for both a VAD and transplant program, to make sure to meet all legal and compliance standards, to hire the necessary administrative and clinical staff, to list patients for transplant, and above all, to hire the right people to lead them through the process, and to help launch a successful program.

Dr. Mike Dickinson, a Grand Rapids native fresh off a cardiology fellowship at Cleveland Clinic, was offered the post of medical director of the transplant program.

"We needed someone with the local connections and knowledge of the organization and its needs," Dickinson said of his decision to accept the post. "What I needed was a surgeon with profound experience to handle all of the things that I couldn't do. To get someone like Asghar was key."

Khaghani arrived with a great deal of fanfare as surgical director in October 2010. Because of his tremendous resume and world renown, many were surprised and delighted to find him to be a humble, down-to-earth, and very approachable person. Following Khaghani's arrival, the team did not have to wait long for its first patient.

In September 2010, 50-year-old West Michigan native Rahn Bentley attended a Grand Rapids Rotary Club luncheon where Rich DeVos shared his experience as a heart transplant recipient and his advocacy for organ donation.

Bentley was more than a curious attendee at the luncheon. He was listed with UNOS, awaiting a donor heart for transplant. Bentley was born with a congenital heart defect and had his first open-heart surgery at age six at Butterworth Hospital. He had undergone four open-heart surgeries, including one earlier in 2010, when doctors installed an LVAD.

In October, UNOS agreed to transfer Bentley's transplant listing from Northwestern Memorial Hospital to Spectrum Health. On November 30, he got the call that would change his life and mark Spectrum Health's first heart transplant case. The operation, led by Dr. Khaghani, lasted about eight hours.

"He got the call at 5 p.m. and was being wheeled into the operating room at 6 p.m.," Bentley's twin brother, Ray Bentley, a former NFL football player and sports broadcaster, told the *Grand Rapids Press*.

"I've played in Super Bowls, and it doesn't even come close to seeing my brother when he woke up yesterday," Bentley said. "We were both crying and holding each other. Our birthday was Thanksgiving, so this was a hell of a present."

Following Bentley's successful surgery, Dickinson says that what really surprised everyone was the rapid flurry of transplants once the program got underway. They discovered that West Michigan had needed a transplant program even more than anticipated.

Following Bentley's successful transplant, they performed one other in the final month of 2010. In 2011, they performed thirteen, nearly a quarter of the fifty-five adult heart transplants undertaken in the state that year. There was enough growth to warrant the addition of a lung transplant program, which got underway in 2013.

By 2015, the team was accounting for more than a quarter of all heart transplants and nearly a third of the lung transplants taking place in Michigan. They had also successfully carried out the only two combined heart/lung transplants in the state dating back more than a dozen years.

The milestones fell one-by-one. In 2015, the team carried out four transplants in a twenty-four-hour period, a marathon and mammoth undertaking for any team, let alone a program that was barely five years old. By late 2017, the team had carried out its hundredth heart and hundredth lung transplant.

Khaghani's presence provided a once-in-a-lifetime training ground in transplant procedures for local cardiothoracic surgeons, including Dr. Boeve, who would succeed Khaghani in 2017.

But Khaghani was still the "Energizer Bunny," as staff affectionately called him, whose seemingly boundless energy set the tone.

"Early on he did back-to-back transplants, two hearts in one day," Dickinson recalled. "I was concerned. Here was a guy who was close to retirement, and transplant is a prolonged process. I went down to recovery and asked him, 'Do you really think this is smart to be doing another transplant?'"

Khaghani's response: "You don't understand—this is such a thrill for me. I love this."

15

The Way Back

To this day, youngest daughter, Jami, remembers the carton of pool water from the Holland Community Aquatic Center that her father kept with him on his nightstand at the hospital… "He liked the smell of it, to be able to focus on something. It could be months or years from now. But that was the goal, to always be back in the pool."

FRED AND JEAN were still in bed when their home phone rang at 7:00 a.m. on Tuesday, June 17, 2014. When they saw the caller ID, they knew that this was "The Call."

"Neither Jean nor I ran to the phone. We just kind of stood there prompting each other to answer the call," Fred said. "It seemed as though time was moving in slow motion. A hundred thoughts flashed through my mind in an instant. Just as the answering machine was responding, I picked up. 'Hello' was the best I could muster."

Gordon was at the farm of his friend Bruce Vartian, watching him move a pile of wood when his call came.

"At that time, I couldn't do squat," Gordon said. "I walked 20 feet from the car to where I was watching Bruce when I got the call from my coordinator, Eric, who said, 'Come in now, have we got a pair for you.' Bruce said, 'Get in my car—we are leaving now.' It was June 17, early in the afternoon."

The moment Gordon, Fred, and their loved ones had been waiting for had finally arrived. If all went well over the next twenty-four hours of organ extraction from the donor and implantation into the recipients—and through the succeeding days and months of recovery and rehabilitation—Fred and Gordon might emerge with renewed vitality and vigor. But what kind of quality of life could Fred and Gordon realistically expect?

THE FIRST HOURS, days, and even months of a heart and lung transplant can be an enormous challenge for both the patient and caregivers.

Both heart and lung transplant patients awaken in a special, sterile transplant ICU, still connected to a ventilator. Once the ventilator is removed, usually within 24 hours, patients remain connected to a variety of monitors and catheters.

If all goes well, much of the remaining 10–14-day hospital stay includes education about recovery, rehabilitation, and immunosuppressant drugs that the patient will take for the rest of his life. Patients are also placed on antibacterial, antifungal, and antiviral medications, which can be altered depending on the progress of recovery.

Beginning in and following their transfer out of ICU, patients receive physical, cardiac, and/or pulmonary therapy every day, all of which is managed by their post-transplantation coordinators.

After discharge, follow-up visits are generally scheduled every one to two weeks for the first several months. If all goes according to plan, these visits can be scaled back to monthly or bi-monthly visits after six months. After a year, visits are generally conducted quarterly. Patients may resume driving a car when the incisions in the sternum heal, and can often return to work several months post-surgery.

Of course, these typical guidelines apply to the "average" patient and do not necessarily take into account episodes of organ rejection or infection, which are quite common.

According to 2017 statistics and information provided by UptoDate, an evidence-based, physician-authored clinical decision support resource, heart transplant recipients:

…have an average of one to three episodes of rejection in the first year after transplantation. Between 50 and 80 percent of people experience at least one rejection episode. Acute rejection is most likely to occur in the first three to six months, with the incidence declining significantly after this time.

In the first year, most deaths are due either to acute rejection (18 percent) or infections (22 percent). Infections often develop as a result of the anti-rejection medications and weakened immune system that are required to prevent rejection…Rejection is less common after the first year, and by four to five years after transplantation, less than 10 percent of deaths are the result of rejection.

For lung recipients, UptoDate reports the following:

Acute allograft rejection is a significant problem in lung transplantation…more than a third of lung transplant recipients are treated for acute rejection in the first year after transplant. Acute rejection is responsible for approximately 4 percent of deaths in the first 30 days following transplantation…Primary graft dysfunction…which occurs in the early hours to days after transplant, is the leading cause of death in the first 30 days after transplantation, accounting for more than 25 percent of deaths.

The long-term prognosis was better for Fred than for Gordon:

The median survival for heart transplants performed between 1982 and June 2015 was 11 years for adult recipients and 16 years for pediatric recipients. Patient survival has steadily improved since the 1980s, with one-year survival rates now exceeding 85 percent for adult patients and 90 percent for pediatric patients.

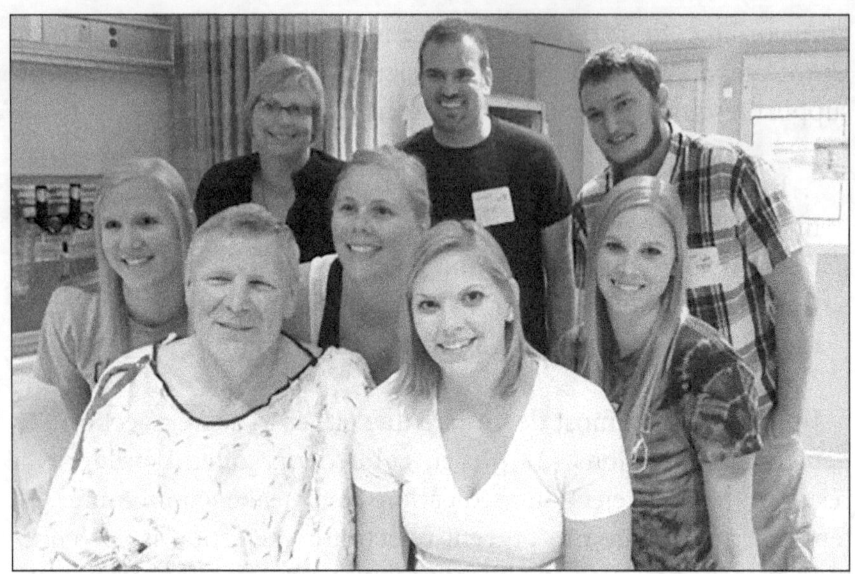

Pre-transplant Nelis family pic

The median survival for all adult (lung) recipients is 6.0 years, but bilateral lung recipients appear to have a better median survival than single lung recipients (7.4 versus 4.6 years, respectively).

FOR JEAN AND the Nelis girls, who were joined by Kelly and Heather's husbands, Ryan Nicholas and Colt Dykstra, and by several family friends, June 18, 2014 was a long night of waiting. They were informed at 4 a.m. that the heart had not yet arrived. At 6 a.m. they were updated that it *still* had not arrived.

"It had been lightning and thundering all night long, so we were a bit concerned that the heart still wasn't there," Jean recalled. "Then about 6:30 a.m., the transplant coordinator, Eric, told us the heart had arrived. We were all elated and cheered."

Then reality crept back in. Jean was nervous thinking about the heart being sewn in and then not starting to beat. What would happen then?

"Close to noon, Dr. Khaghani came and told us that the heart was in and beating and everything had gone great," she remembered. "It was a moment of great relief."

AT NOON ON June 18, Fred was transferred to the ICU on the fifth floor of the center. When his family was finally allowed to see him, they weren't prepared for what awaited them.

He was hooked up to multiple infusion pumps, machines of unknown purpose whirred and beeped throughout the room, and he was still breathing through a respirator, which he later tried to describe to his brood with a swimming metaphor as "fly down and underwater back."

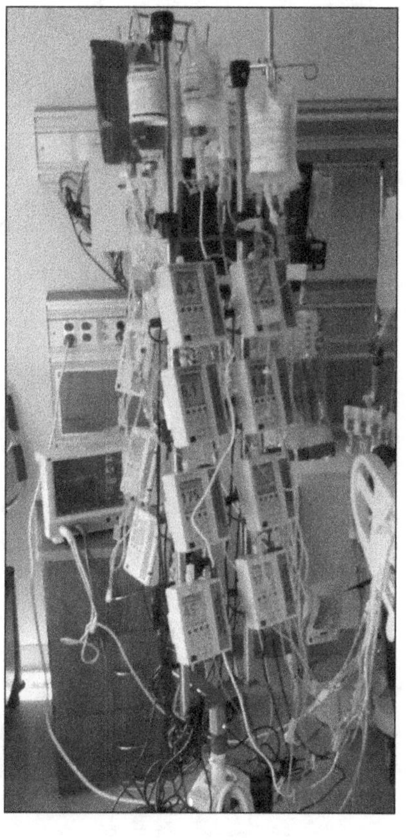

The main shock for Jean and the girls that first day was seeing their husband and father looking so vulnerable.

"His decline almost didn't seem real," said Lindsey. "Most of the time I didn't realize how serious it was because he didn't want us to see him not strong."

But, along with her mother and three sisters, she came face-to-face with that reality on the fifth floor ICU.

"After surgery, there was relief, but it was weird," she added. "There were so many tubes; if you didn't know it was him, you wouldn't recognize him."

"All of us were there," said Heather. "He had tubes and ventilators, and you are holding his hand and it's swollen because he has so many things sticking into it. He had so many medicines on that pole."

But Fred's actions depicted in the opening chapter—his determination to lighten the mood with his game of charades about being hit by a truck, and to provide reassurance by insisting on sitting when the physical therapists arrived later that evening—came as no surprise to his family.

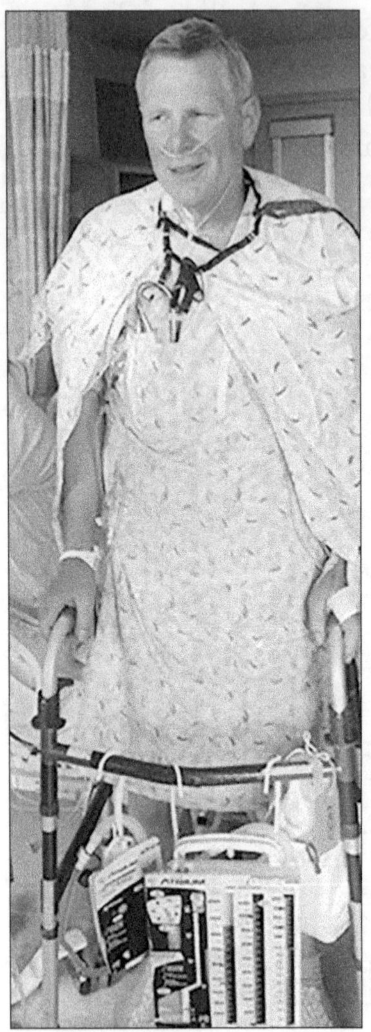

Fred 1st time standing up

"I don't know anybody in my life who works as hard as my dad," says Jami. "He's so mentally disciplined that he puts his mind to something and just does it. His mental fitness was as important as his physical fitness."

For Fred, the hard work would continue over the next months of recovery, but so would the fun—because you can't have one without the other.

"Fred probably has brought more joy to the people at Spectrum Health than anyone," said longtime friend and Dirty Dude, Dr. David Young. "It was absolute lunacy in that room. Fred is crazy, with a very unusual sense of humor, and he had a way to inject something funny no matter how miserable he was feeling," he added.

"Even when he was sick, he cared about giving the nurses and doctors a good day," said Kathryn Olney. "His goal was to make them smile and laugh before they left his room."

On June 20, occupational and physical therapy started in earnest. Fred's therapists wanted him to take deep breaths and blow in the incentive spirometer to keep his lungs clear and prevent pneumonia. He stood and walked and sat in the recliner twice.

"He is tired but just as determined," Jean wrote on Fred's Care Pages digital platform, which was shared with family, friends, and well-wishers.

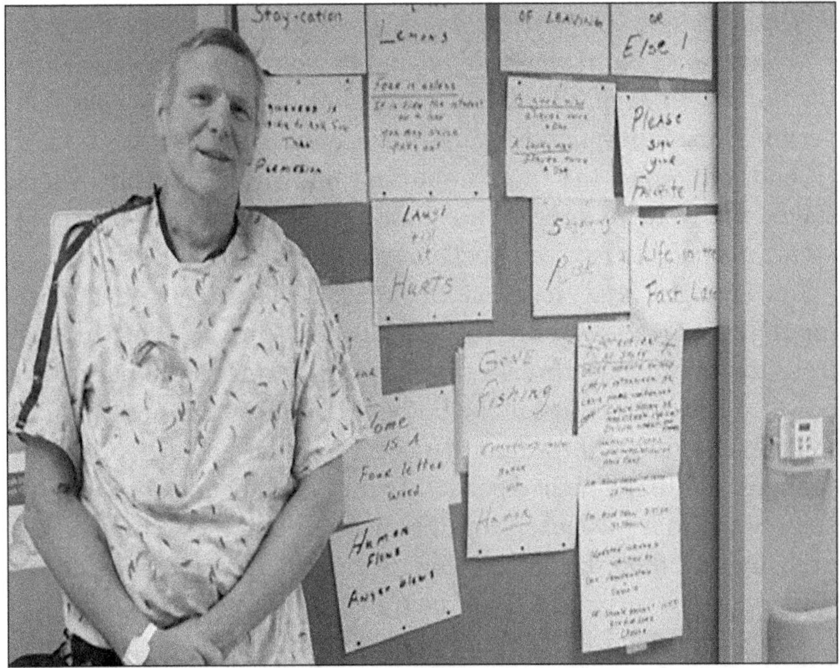

Feeling great after transplant

On post-transplant day four, Fred's doctors began weaning him off some of his IV medications to the oral meds he would take on his return home.

On day five, Fred was moved from the ICU to the 7th floor of the Frederik Meijer Heart Center. He was greeted with a sign on the door of his new room that said, "Welcome Back!!! We Missed You!" signed by his caregivers. He also gained a bit more freedom of movement when a PICC line, an IV access port used for a prolonged period of time, was put in to administer IV med doses, and two arterial lines were removed.

That freedom allowed him to post his own hand-lettered leafs of paper on the door and on the wall of his room with requests for visitors and staff to sign, indicating their favorite saying, slogan, or stray thought.

These included: *Fear is useless. It is like the interest on a loan you may never take out; Lemonade requires lemons; Gone fishing; Life in the fast lane; Laugh 'til it hurts; Forgiveness is easier to ask for than permission;* and *Just another stay-cation,* among others.

And, of course, the most important and most poignant, which stayed affixed to his door for the duration of his stay: *Only the Father knows the balance between grief and gratitude.*

On day eight, Fred's recovery hit a snag. He had surgery that morning to remove the rest of his LVAD driveline, the cable that extends from the pump, out through the skin, and connects the pump to a power source worn outside the body. When the abdominal surgeon went in, he found the surgery was more involved than originally thought. The driveline had partially penetrated the upper part of the colon wall. So it was necessary to remove a bit of the colon with the driveline and then staple the colon. Both Jean and Fred felt that this surgery was more painful than the transplant surgery.

Longtime friend Dr. Steve Van Wylen would call that an understatement, and he believes it's a miracle that Fred didn't die from the penetration of his colon when the driveline was originally placed at the time of the LVAD surgery.

"It is utterly miraculous that he didn't get an infection in the abdominal cavity," Van Wylen said. "Without an operation to fix the perforation it is almost guaranteed that one would develop peritonitis and sepsis. To me, that's something outside of normal physiology," he added. "In his overall weakened state, Fred should have died of an abdominal infection."

Not only did Fred recover from surgery, but on July 2, day fourteen, the results of Fred's first heart biopsy came back showing no sign of rejection, news that the Nelis family was ecstatic to receive. Fred also had his last chest tube and external pacemaker wires removed that morning, and in the afternoon, for physical therapy, he walked up and down a flight of stairs, one of the tests he needed to pass to be able to go home. He was also able to walk without a walker, meaning he was no longer labeled a "fall risk."

As the milestones fell, Fred still had plenty of time on his hands, much of which he spent missing Jean.

"Jean and I have been through a lot of unsavory days," he reflected. "As bad as I felt, she'd walk in the room and I felt better. The longest time at the hospital was when she looked at her watch and said I've got to beat the traffic out of here."

He spent some of that time contemplating the weird numerology surrounding his transplant experience. Fred's cardiomyopathy diagnosis had been made at age 38; he was the 38th heart transplant in Spectrum Health's Richard DeVos Heart and Lung Transplant Program; if you add the numbers representing the date of his transplant (6-18-14), they sum to 38.

Fred said he also had a premonition that his transplant date would be June 21 and that his discharge date would be July 7. Those are special dates for him: his father died on June 21, 2001, and his mother passed away on July 7, 2000.

"I think both my parents were silently attempting to keep my memory of them alive," he later wrote.

The bond between Fred and Jean was strengthened by the care and support he had provided when she had her own health scare. If heart issues occur with frequency in Fred's family, Jean's family has been profoundly impacted by cancer.

Jean's mother, Edith, fell ill on Memorial Day in 1988. The family was at the cottage on Bills Lake when they noticed her acting strangely. In June, she was diagnosed with a brain tumor. Edith responded well to her surgery, which took place in July, but during radiation treatment in August, she developed a fever, which quickly turned into pneumonia, and within three days she died at age 57.

Edith had eleven siblings, including several who died of uterine, colon, and brain cancer. Jean was diagnosed with colon cancer in 2004 at age 44, and previously was diagnosed (at age 38!) with IgA nephropathy, a kidney disease that occurs when an antibody lodges in the kidneys, resulting in inflammation that, over time, may hamper the kidneys' ability to function.

In 2011, Jean underwent genetic testing and was diagnosed with Lynch syndrome, an inherited disorder that increases the risk of many types of cancer, particularly colorectal cancer.

Jean has been cancer-free since 2004, and her kidneys have been stable. At present, she has about 25 percent kidney function, and her goal is to keep stable to avoid a transplant. If it came to that, all three of Jean's siblings, Mike, John, and Gail (none of whom are afflicted with Lynch syndrome), have agreed they would be tested to donate a kidney to their baby sister.

Jean continued to update Fred's Care Pages throughout his recovery. He was indeed scheduled for discharge on July 7, in line with his premonition, but a completely booked cath lab postponed some final tests so they were forced to wait another day. On that day Jean wrote:

"Fred will have the biopsy done in the morning, and then discharge will start. That is a slow process too so hopefully we will be home by dinner! Had a quiet and uneventful weekend, just getting stronger. Fred has been walking quite a bit in the mornings, a mile around the floor for the last 4 days at least."

Fred's walking had not gone unnoticed by others.

"You know when Fred is around, that's for sure," recalled transplant manager Krista Veine. "He is very determined about his goals. Fred always wanted to know if he was the first to do everything—extubated first, the first one to do laps," she added. "Those characteristics can equate to success in a transplant patient."

Gordon also noticed Fred cruising the corridors with his walker, and despite his own misery, the irrepressible extrovert was dying to have someone to talk to. But on July 8, Fred received another setback. On the way to discharge, he breezed through his heart biopsy, chest X-ray, echocardiogram, and EKG. He believed he was set to go home when the doctor came in to inform him that his white blood count and hemoglobin had been too low in the morning's lab work. This required an adjustment of one of his anti-rejection drugs.

The next day, the long-awaited discharge finally took place.

"We sat out on the deck in the sunshine and ate dinner, and it felt really good," wrote Jean. "Now we have to get used to a new medication regime, and get Fred rested and fattened back up!"

GORDON'S TRANSPLANT WAS also a success, although, as a gadget and technology junkie, he says he wishes he'd been able to enjoy checking out the operating room for a bit longer.

"They wheeled me in about 2 a.m. and I'm looking around this place, and I'm just in awe of all of this stuff," he recalled. "I got to enjoy it for about a minute and a half and that was it."

His surgery also was not without complications. Gordon's Alpha-1 had created unnatural scar tissue—adhesions—between the lung and adjacent tissues, which can be difficult to remove. In the course of cutting these adhesions, Gordon experienced a small tear in his aorta that needed to be repaired.

Though Gordon's recollections of his medical procedures are not always the most accurate or reliable, he is always more than happy to share the gory details.

"My aorta had burst, so they opened me up, took out the intestines and the stomach, and used methyl blue to coagulate the blood in the chest cavity so they could vacuum it up," he said. "Afterward, they stitched my aorta back together."

His recovery was also far from easy.

"I went into ICU after the surgery," he recalled. "It took a few days for my head to clear. The drugs used are so powerful, it takes days to recover."

As mentioned earlier, lung transplant recipients often die from pneumonia and infections caused by swallowing food into the lungs, so he was allowed no food or water for three weeks and could not leave his bed for the first week. After three weeks, he had to learn how to swallow again. According to Gordon, he had also developed MRSA in his right lung.

Methicillin-resistant Staphylococcus aureus (MRSA) is a bacterium that causes staph infections and is tougher to treat than most strains of staphylococcus, because of its resistance to commonly used antibiotics. Hazmat suits were required to enter his room, and

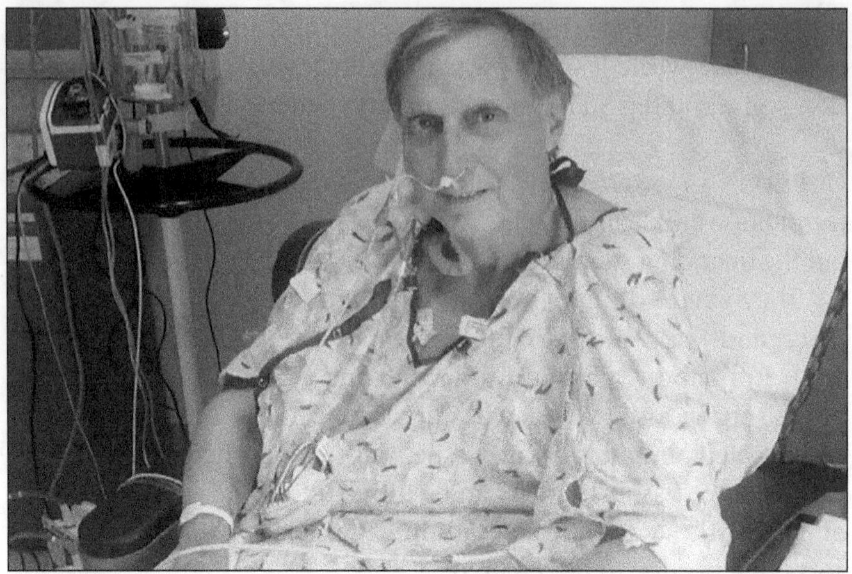

Gordon in hospital bed

he had to remain in the hospital for an entire month until he and the area were declared MRSA-free.

Because Gordon wasn't allowed visitors and couldn't leave his bed, it was a while before he and Fred connected. When he was finally up and about and able to find Fred's room, it turned out to be the day of Fred's LVAD driveline surgery. Their reunion would have to wait for just a while longer.

"As soon as you possibly can, they encourage you to go out walking to keep the suspension of the legs and the gainful use of your stability," he recalled. "The problem I had was that I had bags of stuff and big plastic boxes to collect the drainage. Going out for a walk was a challenge for me, because I had the chest draining box and a Christmas tree full of drugs."

The hospital routine got very old for him in his weeks on 7 Heart.

"They talk about therapeutic sleep, but the interruptions never stop in that place," he grumbled. One perk was his room, however, which had a perfect view of the Fourth of July fireworks celebration over the Grand River in downtown Grand Rapids.

ON JULY 14, Fred had another setback. He awoke with a horrible pain in his right lower leg, which necessitated a return trip to the hospital. The diagnosis was a small blood clot in his leg, for which he was treated with blood thinners to dissolve the clot.

"Please pray for him tonight," Jean wrote in Fred's Care Pages.

Fred was home the next day, though he was required to remain on blood thinners. "What's one more med?" he wrote.

By July 25, he'd had his fourth weekly heart cath with no signs of rejection. More importantly, he was delighted to announce that as soon as the wound in his side closed, it would mean shower and steam room time followed by a return to the pool.

On August 7, he took that next step.

"Not since November 17, 2013 have I had a blissful, enjoyable, wonderful, sweet, hot, long, power shower," he wrote. "For the last 8½ months the bird bath had to suffice."

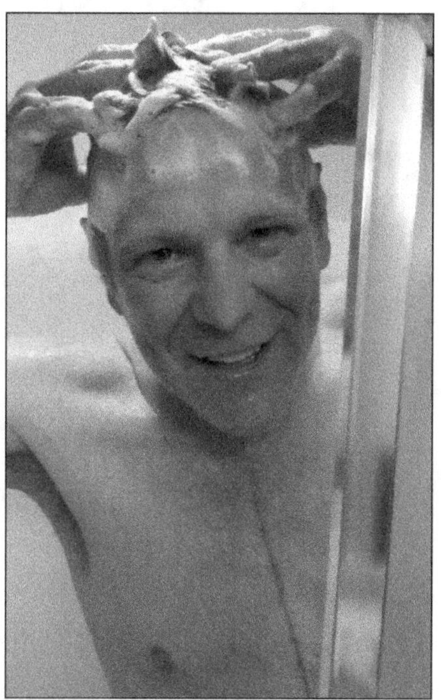

Fred 1st shower

The picture he posted to his Care Pages depicts a look of sheer bliss. But if the shower was delightful, his first dip in the pool, a week later on August 14, was a cross between Christmas and the first day of vacation.

"This week was marvelous," he wrote. "Had my first shower, went back into the steam room, and had a swim Friday p.m. and Saturday a.m. (1600 yds)."

To this day, youngest daughter, Jami, remembers the carton of pool water from the Holland Community Aquatic Center that her father kept with him on his nightstand at the hospital.

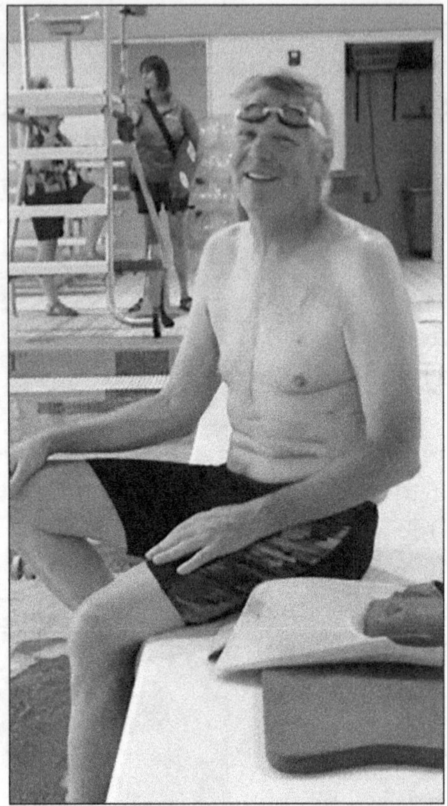

Fred's first swim after surgery

"That was the goal from the start—to always be able to come back and swim," Jami said. "He liked the smell of it, to be able to focus on something. It could be months or years from now. But that was the goal, to always be back in the pool."

In fifty-seven days post-surgery, Fred had met that goal. To have that experience, to feel his body slice through the water—that might have been enough for some people.

However, even then, just a day after his first shower in more than eight months, Fred's competitive edge shines just perceptibly through the fog of his bliss.

"It is going to take a while to get back to JV status," he wrote. "Guess time is what I have a lot of these days."

16

It's a Wonderful Life

"Just a couple of days ago I came out of Memorial Medical in Ludington, after giving a blood draw, and there was a guy who was much younger than I was with his oxygen bottle leaning up against a post trying to collect his breath enough to make it the rest of the way, and I thought, 'Oh my God, don't ever forget that. That's where I used to rest, that's where I used to stop and try to get things under control so that when you walked up to the doors you didn't look like you were going to fall apart.'"

—Gordon Veldman

FRED'S HOMECOMING was a joyous one. He was surrounded by the love of his wife, daughters, and a young grandson, Blake, as well as the support of his siblings, extended family, and friends. It was a time of sharing and thanksgiving, but also a time of celebration.

In August, on the two-month anniversary of Fred and Gordon's successful transplant surgeries, Fred and Jean traveled up the coast to Pentwater to meet with Gordon, who had been home for about

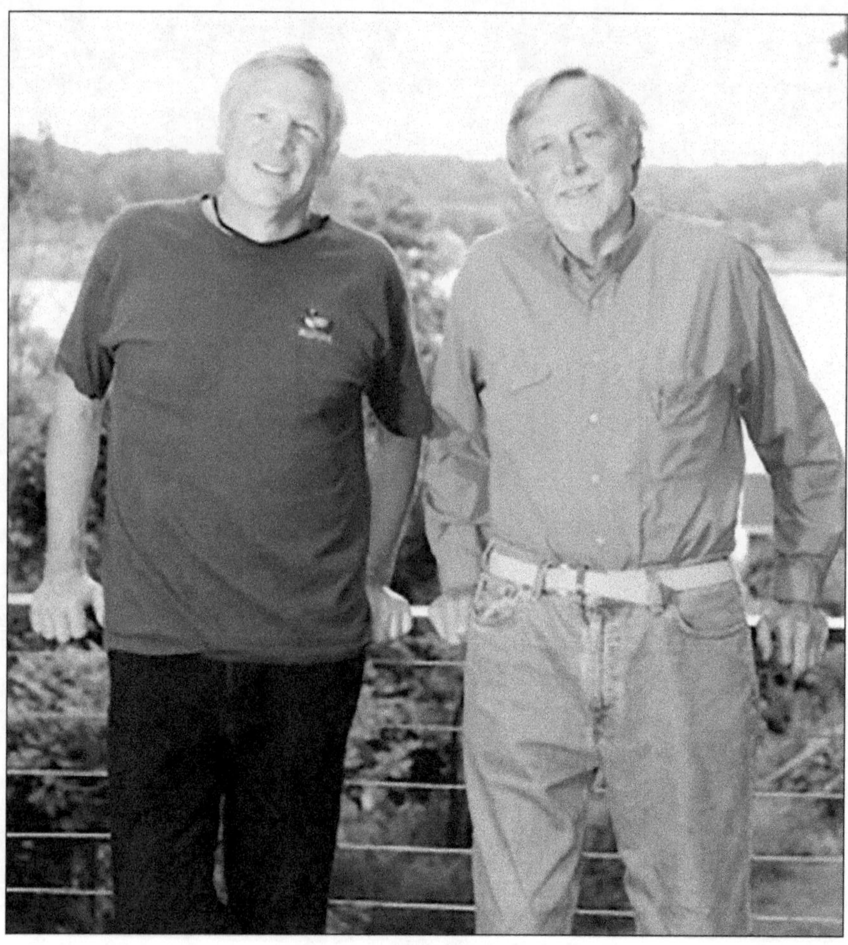

The transplant brothers

a week. Gordon's friend, Joe Clark, took a photo of the Transplant Brothers and professionally mounted and framed it for each of them, and for display in the waiting room of the Richard DeVos Heart and Lung Transplant Clinic.

Fred felt well enough in September to gather the Dirty Dudes and Dusty Dames up north at Black Mountain Lodge. The trip was a sold-out success with all of the regulars, as well as the not-so-regulars, in attendance to welcome Fred back to the fold.

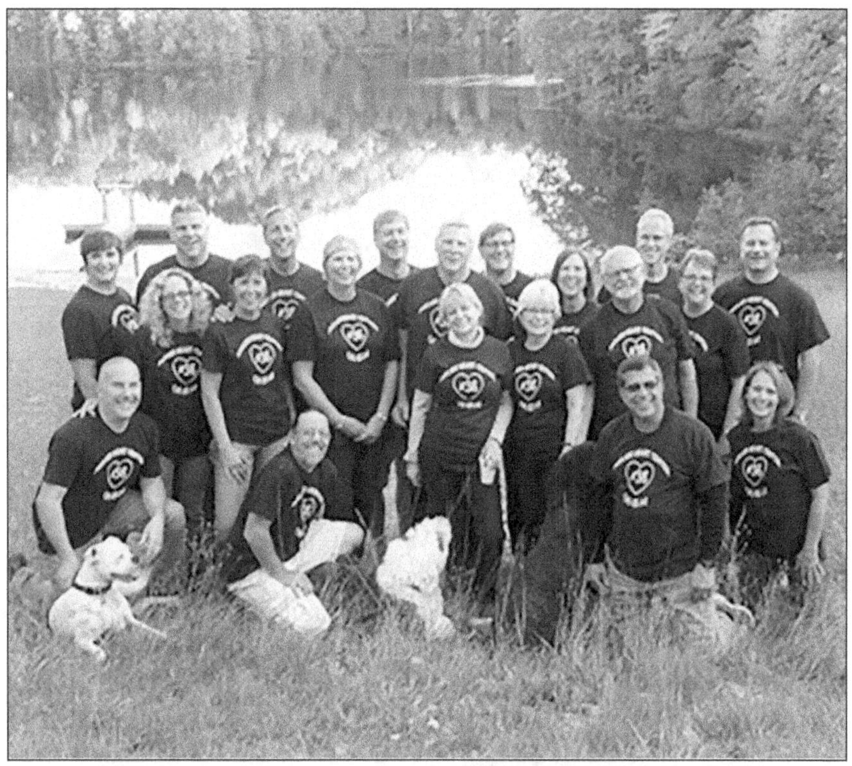

Group Picture at Black Mtn Lodge

The group decided on one final quadding adventure the first week-end in October. Upon his return home from "an awesome weekend quadding, eating, socializing up north, and feeling fine," Fred found an urgent message from the hospital on his answering machine: his white blood cell count, especially his neutrophil levels, were very low. He was directed to report to isolation at the hospital, where he spent four days having his meds adjusted.

He quickly stabilized, however, and by the end of the month was able to reduce some of his medications when his biopsy reported no evidence of rejection for the eighth straight time. He was feeling well enough to host a Halloween party where he introduced Gordon as the guest of honor to the friends who had not yet met him.

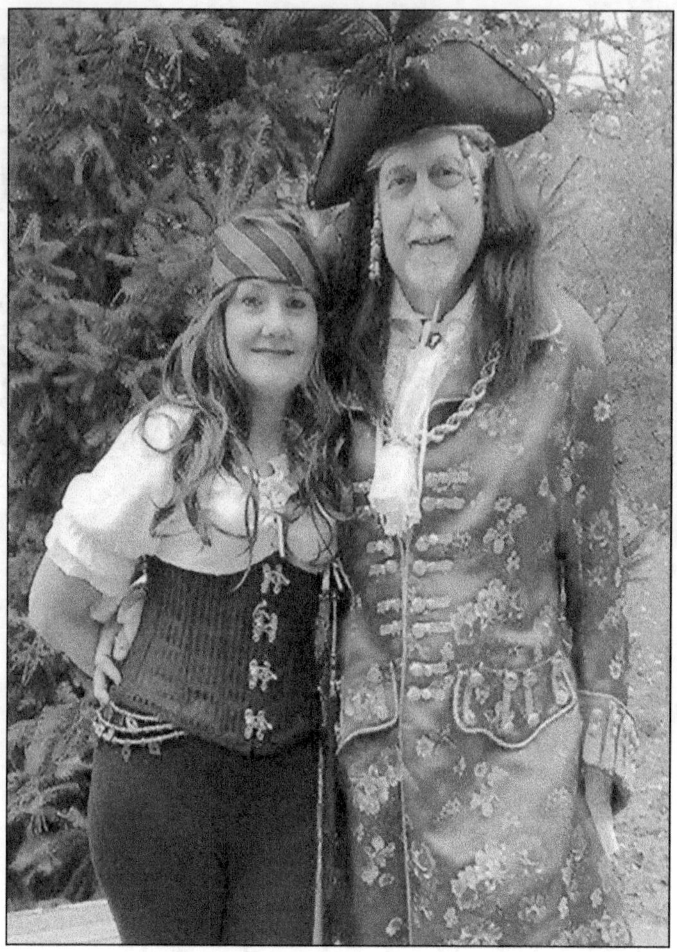

Gordon & Nancy Halloween party

GORDON'S HOMECOMING, MEANWHILE, had been a lonely and dispiriting one.

His girlfriend, Barbara, lived in Grand Rapids, close to the hospital, whereas Gordon lived ninety minutes away. Although she had her hands full caring for her ailing mother, she took on the significant responsibility of being Gordon's caregiver for a couple of weeks, serving as a "halfway house" during his convalescence, before his return home to Pentwater.

Later, he remembered: "When Barbara dropped me off after the care-giver routine, I just unloaded the car and carried it in and thought, 'I'm really no further along than I was before. Why did I go through this?'"

Then, within weeks, everything changed. At age 66, Gordon met a woman who threw his heart for a loop.

"Then I met Nancy and it all became very clear," he recalled. "I never dreamed it could be a possibility."

Nancy Zielinski was a recently widowed Chicagoan, an accountant and financial manager whose husband George had died of heart failure in 2013. The couple began visiting Pentwater in the late 1960s and had bought frontage on Lake Michigan in 1976. Throughout the years, they constructed a dwelling they used as a summer cottage. When they retired, they refurbished the cottage, turning it into a year-round home. They moved to Pentwater permanently in 2006. Although the couple was married for more than forty years, Nancy describes it as a lonely, unhappy and, at times, abusive marriage.

"I fell head over heels with Gordon by mid-October 2014," Nancy recalled. "I had found my soulmate."

For soulmates they had a hell of a time getting together, though. For one thing, Gordon was still in a relationship with Barbara, and for another, events seemed to conspire against them every time they tried to connect.

Nancy recalls that she first met Gordon in March 2014, about three months prior to his transplant. Gordon never refers to this meeting, though, either not remembering or preferring to place their meeting after his transplant. He had already been listed for transplant and was at an all-time, physical low point.

"Maybe he didn't want me to know him then," Nancy says.

She recalls that they met at the Artisan Learning Center in Pentwater, where he was in the process of donating a lot of the wood, metal-working materials, and other tools he had accumulated and stored over the years—giving away his possessions in preparation for death.

"When he needed to be there, he got there early so people wouldn't see him struggle," she said.

Although Gordon may not remember, Nancy says he did try to call her in April.

The house that Nancy and George built for their retirement stands on a lonely dead-end street less than fifty yards from the shore of Lake Michigan. It is a gorgeous and enviable location in the summer. During a winter storm, however, high winds, waves, and flying snow and ice can make things dicey. It is common to lose power. In April, a storm with high winds was forecast and Nancy was afraid she might be stuck. Her friends, Ted and Joan Cuchna, invited her to stay at their house, closer to town.

Gordon found out from Ted Cuchna that Nancy would be staying there, so he called her there to ask her to dinner, leaving a message on the Cuchnas' answering machine. Nancy, meanwhile, had decided to go back to her house when the winds died down and never received the message.

"He never heard from me and must have figured I wasn't interested," Nancy recalled. "That bothered me all summer."

It's not quite a pre-cellphone anecdote, but it might as well be. Meanwhile, Gordon had other, more immediate concerns that summer, such as recovering from his date with destiny on June 18, 2014.

The two finally managed to spend time together in September. Nancy wanted to get rid of a hot tub and wooden slats for a deck she and her late husband had bought forty years ago, and after all this time she had no intention of installing them. She asked Ted Cuchna to dispose of the hot tub and either deliver the slats to the Artisan Center or take them to burn in his wood stove.

On the same day, Gordon called Ted asking to borrow a reciprocating saw so he could cut up and dispose of his own hot tub. Ted saw an opportunity to play matchmaker.

"Ted asked Gordon if he was going to get another hot tub," Nancy said. "And when Gordon said he planned to, Ted told him, 'Well, I've got one in the truck you can use.'"

The hot tub happened to be missing a few pieces that were still back at Nancy's house. So one thing led to another, and by late fall,

Gordon was reciprocating Nancy's sentiments and sharing the same thoughts.

"I can't be without her anymore," he said, referring to Nancy. "It's the most revealing thing—to finally get to the point where that song 'I Want to Know What Love Is' has colored itself and become reality. I've finally got something that I admired in couples."

His lung capacity was also rapidly improving, allowing him to re-enter a world from which his disease had forced him to retreat. From his pre-transplant FEV1 measurement of 23 percent, he had jumped to an FEV1 of 93 percent in August, and by fall he was at 100 percent.

"To be at the brink of death—to see your dying in your friends' faces—is an unforgettable experience," Gordon said. "And to be here today, able to walk, run, bike, able to do the things I never thought I would do again, is a continual miracle.

"And best of all, Nancy finally gets a chance to sit in that hot tub she's owned for forty years," he added.

His boundless energy was vintage Gordon, and impressive for a man half his age. With the time, means, and finally his health on their hands, Gordon and Nancy set out on a whirlwind courtship that included constant activity and plans to travel the world.

"I say to him, 'I wish I had met you earlier,'" Nancy says. "I suddenly have all this attention and it is very flattering to me. I always feel very loved. His face lights up and he says, 'Oh, Nancy, I am so glad you are here.' Who wouldn't like that?"

New Year's Eve brought travel plans for both couples. Fred and Jean traveled to Florida, staying at Marathon Key with their daughters and their spouses.

Gordon and Nancy, meanwhile, spent New Year's Eve in downtown Chicago at a boutique hotel, dining one evening at The Walnut Room, which was decorated spectacularly for the holidays. While in her hometown, Nancy took the opportunity to introduce her new beau to her sisters and several cousins and aunts. When they returned to Pentwater, Gordon declared it "the best honeymoon I ever had!"

The next month, the couple ventured a bit farther afield with a West Coast trip that included flying into Las Vegas and renting a Pontiac Firebird for the drive to California. While there, they visited Nancy's aged parents in Hemet, along with the Salton Sea and Joshua Tree National Park. On the way back to Vegas, they drove through a small section of Route 66, at times getting the Firebird up to 120 miles per hour.

"On the West Coast trip, my dad fell in love with Gordon," Nancy recalled. "He wanted to adopt him and vice versa. That is our excuse for not marrying—because we would be brother and sister." (In actuality, Gordon is still married to Beverly, although they have a legal separation.)

Back home in Pentwater, the couple spent some early spring mornings with Gordon's friends Bruce and Ellen Vartian on their wooded property boiling maple syrup.

"Rum and syrup on a cold March morning," Nancy says wistfully. "I would sooner do that than fly to France—the maple boiling, the syrup boiling. It is something else."

THAT SAME MONTH, Fred and Gordon readied themselves to announce their unique story to the public. Plans for a press conference had been in the works for several months but were put on hold because of travel conflicts. As the promise of spring dawned in the northern woods, the Transplant Brothers, as they would soon be dubbed, prepared to step out onto a wider stage to share their story.

On the morning of Monday, March 9, 2015, nine months following their successful transplants, I had the opportunity to meet Fred and Gordon, as well as Jean and Nancy, through my work in media relations and communications for Spectrum Health. As we chatted through the pre-press conference procedures, Gordon was high energy, high spirits, and high fives, while the ever-smiling Fred was a bit more laid back and reserved. I made the mental note that the gregarious Gordon might make a better TV and radio interview, while the thoughtful Fred might work better with the print media.

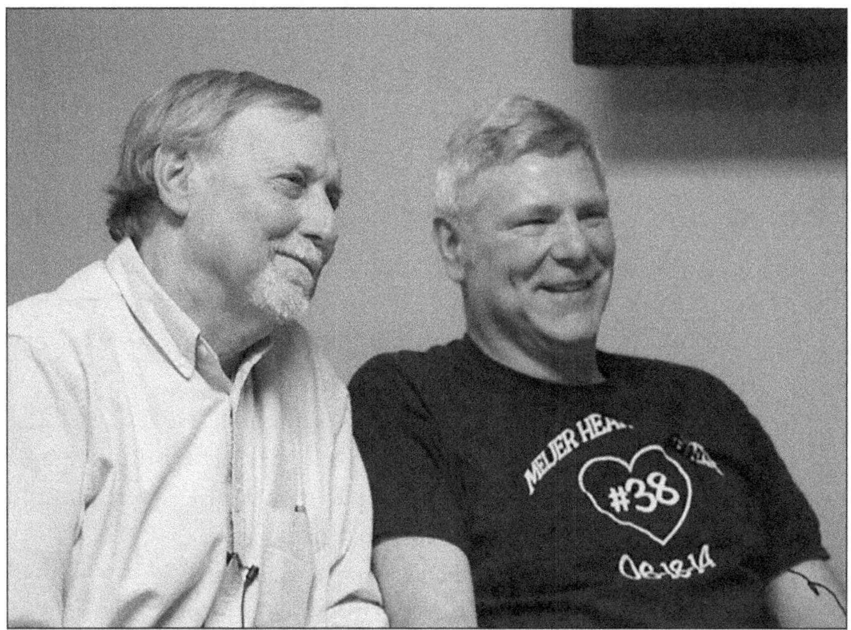

Press Day-Gordon & Fred

I did not yet know their complete back stories or the health struggles they had faced for two decades, only the basics of their diseases and that they were two old friends who had received organs from the same donor on the same night unbeknownst to one another. That type of PR gold was all I needed to know for the time being as we made our way into a conference room crowded with local media. Reporters from the local FOX, NBC, ABC, and PBS affiliates were on hand, along with several radio journalists and Sue Thoms, the longtime health reporter for the *Grand Rapids Press*.

Gordon and Fred sat together at the far end of a long conference room table, and after a brief introduction, the members of the press crowded around and began asking questions about their experiences and the remarkable coincidence that brought them together on the night of June 18, 2014.

Gordon was instantly quotable, as Thoms notes in her story:

"We feel very strongly about the importance of those internal organs and how they support us in our endeavors," he said. "Without them, we are has-beens. Memories.

"Because someone said 'yes,' I've got a future. It's as simple as that," he added.

"My biggest problem was coming to the realization that in order for me to proceed at a quality of life and eventually be free of mechanical and electronic support, somebody had to die," he said.

"It's kind of a deep moral dilemma," he continued. "We are very fortunate that someone's family was so gracious."

What was most noticeable about both men, however, was the buoyancy in their step, their easy camaraderie, their humility and gratitude, but also their eagerness to get on with life, to make the most of their gift, and to make up for lost time.

"The journey gets to begin all over again," Fred said.

"This is going to be a really wonderful summer compared to last summer," Gordon concluded.

The men were giddy as they walked out of the press conference, posed for photos, and prepared to go out to lunch together with the women in their lives. Little did they realize that the media frenzy was just beginning.

Their story was quickly picked up by the Associated Press and published throughout the country and internationally in the *Arizona Republic, Charlotte Observer, Daily Mail, Detroit Free Press, Detroit News, Houston Chronicle, Kansas City Star, Miami Herald, Milwaukee Journal Times, Modesto Bee, MSN.com, Newsday, San Francisco Chronicle,* and *St. Louis Post Dispatch*, to name just a few.

Soon, interview requests were pouring in from ABC News Radio, CBS News, FOX News, and newspapers and TV and radio stations throughout the US and Canada. The photo of the pair taken by Joe Clark made its way around the world.

Gordon's concern that "When the shared transplant with Fred happened, I thought…it can't just be a secret story between two old guys" would prove unnecessary, as the two men found themselves besieged by requests for interviews and personal appearances.

"When that ball started rolling, I thought, 'This is really cool,'" Gordon reflected later. "We've all had experiences in our lives that define us. Here was another opportunity presenting itself for us to stand up and speak when it mattered."

Profiles of the two men continued to appear for the next several weeks, and they were called upon to share their story once again to a rapt crowd at the 2015 Richard DeVos Heart and Lung Transplant Program Celebration of Life, an annual gathering of recipients, donors, families, and care providers.

At the Celebration of Life, Fred shared his Ten Thoughts from My Stryker Bed, a mixture of comedic comments and philosophical insights that included:

Ever wonder why rejection drugs are administered with elbow length rubber gloves, and the patient is told they are good for you?

Courage isn't only found on the battlefield. Often it is found with the quiet resolve that 'tomorrow I will try again.'

The longest hours are spent by family and friends in the waiting rooms.

The scars from transplant are a reminder of the generous gift of a donor and their family.

The best way to improve one's mood is to improve others' moods first.

My hope is that all of us wake up each morning with the excitement and anticipation of a child on Christmas Day. So live boldly, explore new things, and seek out adventure!

Slight variation on one of my favorite movies, *Field of Dreams*: if you build it "they will come" (transplant recipients); instead of "he will come." I think we are soon going to need a bigger venue for our Celebration of Life.

ONE TRAGIC EVENT, however, cast a pall over the excitement of the media frenzy and served as a reminder of the fragility of life and the importance of family (though for Fred and Gordon, this reminder hardly seems necessary).

On the morning of March 11, Fred, Jean, Gordon, and Nancy drove to Grand Rapids for a lengthy, in-depth interview with WOOD Radio, the talk radio market leader in the region. The two couples had prepared for a day of dining out, sightseeing, and shopping, when their plans were cut short by the news that Fred's nephew, Charlotte Nelis's son, had been killed the night before in the line of duty.

US Marines Staff Sgt. Andrew Seif had joined the Marine Corps after graduating from West Ottawa High School in 2006. He served as a combat engineer based out of Camp Pendleton and Twentynine Palms, California from 2006 until 2009. He then joined Marine Special Operations Command (MARSOC) based out of Camp Lejeune, North Carolina, where he lived with his wife, Dawn, who was four months pregnant with their first child. During his nine years in the Marine Corps, he served one tour of duty in Iraq and two tours in Afghanistan.

On the night of March 10, a Black Hawk helicopter carrying Andrew, six other special operations Marines, and four National Guard soldiers crashed in dense fog during a training mission off the coast of Northern Florida. All eleven men were killed.

Andrew had been awarded the Silver Star, just four days prior, for his actions of aiding a wounded team member under heavy fire in Afghanistan in 2012. Fred and Jean would join Charlotte and other family members for his burial at Arlington National Cemetery in April.

JUST AFTER RETURNING from the service for Andrew, Fred suffered the first of two, brief, rejection episodes.

"I knew something was wrong in DC when we walked the Mall and afterward, back in the hotel, I'm taking off my socks and my ankles were three times normal size," Fred said. "My ankles never went down."

Termed an "R2 Event," the episode did not require hospitalization, but Fred was put on 100 milligrams of Prednisone, an oral steroid used for suppressing the immune system, for three days, and on half doses for an additional three weeks.

"I was so on edge from the steroid I couldn't sleep," Fred recalled.

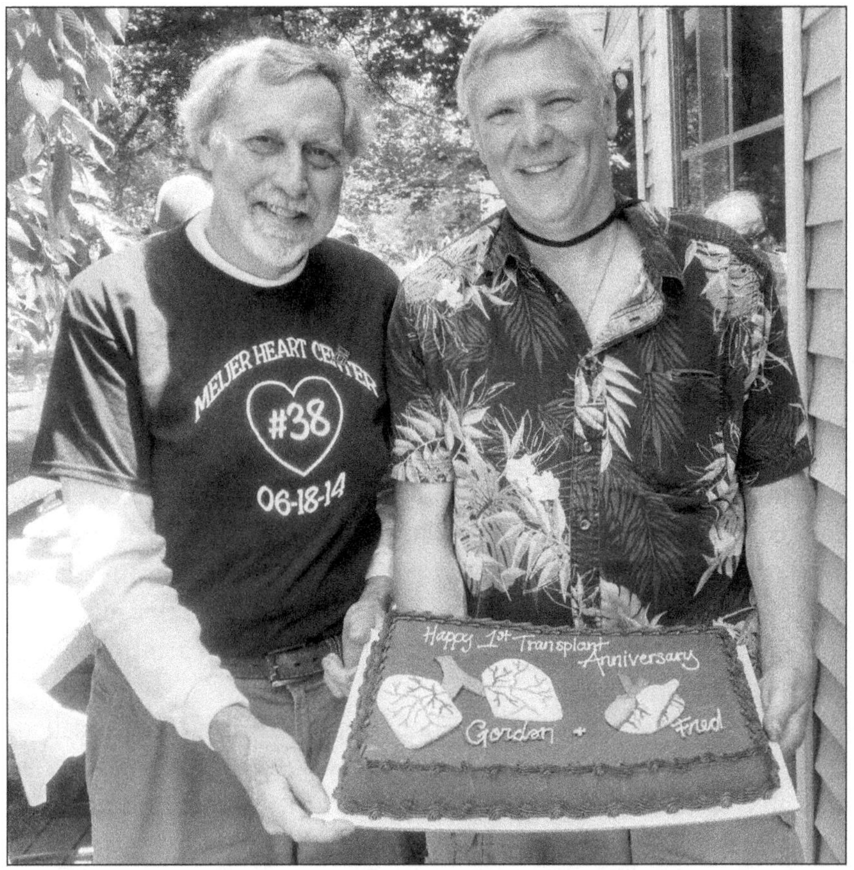

1st year anniversary

It was during those sleepless nights that Fred wrote his Ten Thoughts from My Stryker Bed. But after a full recovery, he was soon preparing for a summer that, according to Gordon's prediction, was "going to be a really wonderful summer compared to last summer."

It had already been a blessed and eventful 2015 for Fred and Jean. In February, daughter Kelly and her husband, Ryan, had welcomed Luke, their second child and Fred and Jean's second grandchild. In addition to this mixture of blessings and tragedy, the year would bring a number of adventures and at least one misadventure.

In June, Fred and Jean held two celebrations of the one-year anniversary of the transplant: a private one, which consisted of a swim for the couple, and a very public party at their house with a multitude of friends and family, including Gordon and Nancy.

It was September, however, that really capped off an eventful summer and set the tone for an even more eventful 2016 to come.

After a six-hour drive one Saturday that month, Fred and Jean arrived at Turkey Run State Park in rural central Indiana for a family reunion on Jean's side. They soon realized that Fred had forgotten his anti-rejection drug.

Jean's brother, Mike, a retired pharmacist, drove them to Crawfordsville, the nearest town of any size, in search of a pharmacy that might be open and able to fill Fred's prescription. Fred repeatedly tried to make contact with Dr. Lee, the on-call physician back at Spectrum Health, but the calls either failed or were immediately dropped due to spotty cellphone coverage. Dr. Lee finally suggested that the best course of action would be for Fred to return to Holland for his meds.

"Needless to say, Dr. Lee was not happy with me," Fred recalled. But finally, a solid telephone connection was established and Dr. Lee was able to talk the young pharmacist through the preparation of Fred's prescription.

Immediately following their return from the reunion, Jean flew to Boston where daughter Jami was finishing a travel nursing contract. Mother and daughter spent a few days together in Boston and then drove back to Michigan. Their trip marked another milestone for Fred.

"This was the first time since the transplant that Jean left me alone to fend for myself for a few days," he recalled, grateful that the time alone was notable for its lack of drama.

Fred was also spending time at Yost Vises discussing the transition from the company's traditional manufacturing business model to expanding e-commerce opportunities. The wind-down of domestic production was slowly being offset by products from offshore producers. It was a crucial time for the business which saw explosive growth in its e-commerce business.

When Jean and Jami returned from Boston, the entire family flew out to Denver for the Great American Beer Festival, where Heather's husband, Colt Dykstra, Head Brewer for Arcadia Brewing, was representing the company. During the visit, Lindsey's boyfriend, Sergio Rocafort, proposed to her in front of the whole family on the 18th tee at Red Rocks Country Club.

"Luckily for everyone, she said yes," Fred mused.

2015 WOULD END on two entirely different notes for Fred and Gordon.

Gordon had indeed spent a much better summer than the previous. Together with Nancy, he had spent the summer months traveling, sailing, visiting friends, and reveling in physical activities that had eluded him for years.

He shared the following anecdote at dinner one night that summer with Fred and Jean and Nancy:

"Just a couple of days ago I came out of Memorial Medical in Ludington after giving a blood draw, and there was a guy who was much younger than I was with his oxygen bottle leaning up against a post trying to collect his breath enough to make it the rest of the way, and I thought, 'Oh my God, don't ever forget that,'" he said.

"That's where I used to rest, that's where I used to stop and try to get things under control so that when you walked up to the doors you didn't look like you were going to fall apart," he added.

The observation seemed to spur him on to even more activity. Trips that summer included a very special weekend on Mackinac Island and sailing around the Great Lakes.

To celebrate Gordon's one-year transplant anniversary, he and Nancy decided to splurge on a stay at Mackinac Island's Grand Hotel. The historic landmark, built in 1873, contains 393 rooms, of which no two are exactly alike, and is renowned for its old-world hospitality and charm. The hotel served as the filming location for *Somewhere in Time*, the 1980 film starring Jane Seymour and Christopher Reeve,

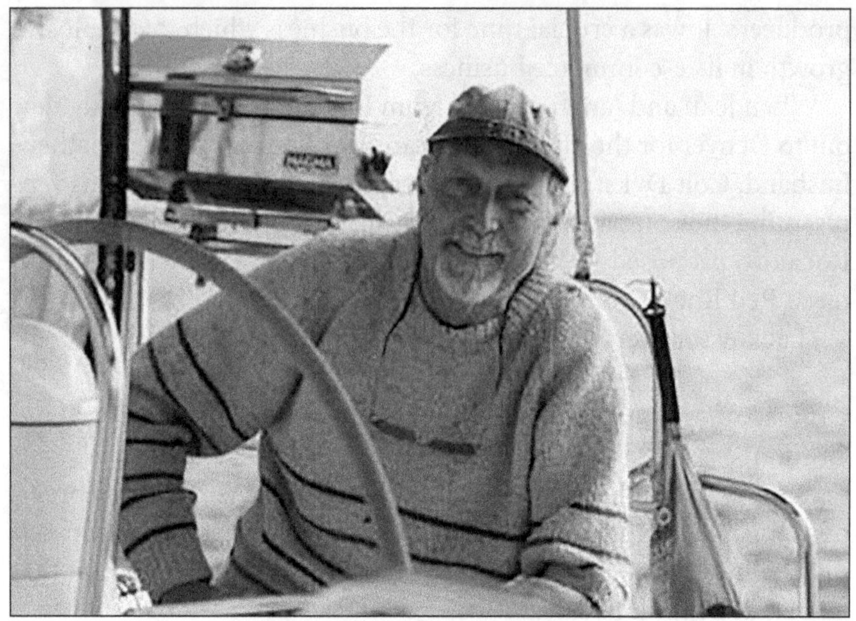

Gordon sailing in North Channel

and has been named by the National Trust for Historic Preservation as "One of a Dozen Distinctive Destinations."

"I had never been there, so we told them we were celebrating the one-year anniversary of a double lung transplant and asked for a room on the bay," Nancy said. "They didn't promise anything, but when we arrived, we were given the room next to the Presidential Suite!"

The couple enjoyed the island's scenic charms, did a lot of walking (there are no motorized vehicles allowed on the island), and bicycled around its eight-mile perimeter.

"That's how well he was," Nancy recalled later. "Gordon had no problems with the bicycle, but I sure did."

On Labor Day, along with three friends, the couple drove up to Gore Bay, Ontario, on Manitoulin Island, where they had rented a 39-foot sailboat to once again sail the North Channel of Lake Huron. On the day they were to set sail, Gordon was moving the outboard motor into the dinghy when he lost his balance and fell into the bay. The motor sank to the bottom, and as it was raining and getting dark, they had to postpone their departure. The next morning, however, the sun broke through and Gordon was able to dive down and retrieve it.

"The rest of the time was beautiful weather," said Nancy. "It was a wonderful, wonderful trip. I remember watching the International Space Station through the porthole of the cabin."

I ran into the couple several times that summer at the hospital. Gordon's stride was lengthy and purposeful, and he was buzzing with energy. He took the time to stop one afternoon to share his frustration with what he considered to be his doctors' short and chafing leash.

The crux of the matter was that he was trying to plan a trip with Nancy to New Zealand for several months during the winter, and he was displeased that his physicians advised against the idea.

Gordon's pulmonologist, Dr. Reda Girgis, medical director of Spectrum Health's lung transplant program, had recommended placing him on Alpha-1 replacement therapy post-transplant. Many experts recommend this therapy, which uses a naturally occurring enzyme to target inflamed tissue caused by the disease.

"We wanted to put him on that for many months, but he didn't want to do it because of cost," said Girgis. "I don't think he even pursued it to see what his out-of-pocket costs would be."

Girgis was also concerned with something that was beginning to show up in Gordon's tests: suspected atypical compliance with his drug regimen.

Thus far, Gordon's cavalier attitude toward taking his meds had yet to cause a problem, but by the end of 2015, things would come to a head for Gordon, who would suffer an acute rejection crisis.

MEANWHILE, FRED CONTINUED his almost religious devotion to his medication regimen. He was training more than ten hours per week and his swim times were beginning to finally show improvement. He was beginning to believe that he might really one day be able to not only participate, but perhaps even compete in some sort of meaning-ful swim competition.

In November, he and Jean attended the Indiana High School Class AAAA Championship Football Game at Lucas Oil Stadium in Indianapolis, in which his twin nephews, the sons of his sister Mary, played key roles in their team's victory.

He thought about his football glory days. He thought about his swimming glory days.

The competitive juices started flowing and he smiled at Jean.

2016 was going to be a very interesting year.

17

Saving the Transplant Games

"Even if you don't meet your particular organ recipient, you feel the love from the other recipients. You feel your loved one did not die in vain."

—Kathy Vogelsang

HOLLY WERLEIN was a healthy young college student who had been named Top Female Athlete of her high school in Gaylord, Michigan, where she swam, played volleyball, and ran track. When she was struck by acute fulminant liver failure that required a transplant in 2004, it was the last thing she ever expected, and there were moments when she didn't know how to continue.

"The first year was definitely rocky," she said. "At first, I couldn't walk very far. I remember thinking, 'This is my life, I'm twenty-one and I had no idea what my life was going to be like.' I knew nobody who had a transplant," she said.

However, in the depths of her despair, she was thrown a much-needed lifeline by an organization she had, heretofore, known nothing about: the US Transplant Games.

"Finding these games gave me the drive to want to be healthy and active," she said. It also put her in touch with an entire community of athletes—living donors, donor families, and recipients—who understood her concerns.

The US Transplant Games (now known as The Transplant Games of America), launched in 1990 and hosted every two years by a different city in the United States, is an Olympics-style event for all organ recipients, with education activities and programs for recipients, living donors, and family members of deceased donors. Hosted in even years, it alternates with the World Transplant Games, held in odd years.

THE US TRANSPLANT Games were the brainchild of National Kidney Foundation Vice President and Regional Director Gary Green. Green developed and grew the program over twenty years, with support from Sandoz, the predecessor company to Novartis Pharmaceuticals, to include more than 6,000 recipients, donor family members, living donors, and medical professionals.

However, in May 2011, the National Kidney Foundation (NKF) announced it would not hold the event in 2012, citing the organization's financial troubles and a change in its strategic scope. The NKF said the Games cost near $3 million to operate—unaffordable at the time, with the country awash in the 2007–2009 financial crisis. The 2010 Games in Madison, Wisconsin, would likely be the last of their kind.

This announcement threw the transplant community into turmoil, with many expressing outrage in the media and on social media. It was akin to the International Olympic Committee announcing that it would no longer organize the Olympics.

T. J. Maciak, a Flint native and Hudsonville, Michigan, resident, decided to do something about it. That same summer of 2011, Maciak, a two-time kidney recipient and transplant games athlete, approached the West Michigan Sports Commission, a non-profit organization in Grand Rapids, to see what could be done to save the games.

The commission was impressed by Maciak's presentation and his passion for keeping the games alive. And, in another moment of serendipity, the Sports Commission happened to include a member who might know just how to make things happen.

Bill Ryan is president of Ryan Marketing Group Technologies, a Grand Rapids-based marketing consulting firm specializing in large-scale events that has been producing the NCAA Men's Basketball Tournament since 1987. Ryan's group had the obvious know-how: In 2011, they were coming off huge wins with record-breaking attendance. Bill Ryan also has skin in the game that helped him to understand Maciak's passion.

The West Michigan Sports Commission announced its support of the 2012 Games at a press conference held on August 23, 2011. The Commission had decided to take on the 2012 Games as a stop-gap measure. Beyond 2012, it was not clear what the future would hold for the games.

Bill Ryan was in attendance to lend support to the board's decision and happened to make the offhand remark that it was also his daughter's birthday. Michelle Ryan would have been 43 that day—had she not been killed in a car accident in 1986 and become a multiple organ donor at the age of 18.

The outpouring of community support was immediate, and Ryan was tapped to lead the organizing committee.

"I was offered the position of chair of the Grand Rapids Games," Ryan said. "But I didn't want an honorary title. I wanted to produce the event. It turned out to be the second largest games ever held—far beyond what we had originally expected."

But that didn't happen without a lot of work and the support of the entire community. Ryan and West Michigan had only one year to organize and put on the games, a process that is traditionally spread across two years after a city is named host site. In the case of the 2012 Games, there were no other cities stepping forward with bids—there was only Grand Rapids.

"Nobody in the professional event world would ever take on a task of that magnitude with less than a year's planning," Ryan said. "We were reprinting signs and banners right up to the start of the Games because we were bringing on new sponsors so late in the game."

"Everything was a volunteer effort," Ryan recalled. "You usually don't find that level of support from a host community. I think it is a sign of what Grand Rapids and the West Michigan community is all about."

Despite the success, the future of the games remained unclear.

"I pushed the group and asked, 'What are we going to do with these games when we are done?'" Ryan said. "As we pushed through the planning and execution of the event, it became obvious that if we didn't step in and do something, the games were going to die after 2012."

So Ryan put together a board of directors and formed a 501(c)(3) called The Transplant Games of America—to continue running the games beyond 2012. Like a lot of non-profits, Ryan's group is under-staffed and underfunded. The games share a headquarters and staff with Ryan Marketing Group Technologies in Grand Rapids.

"It was not our intention to continue that arrangement indefinitely," Ryan said. "But these games would not survive otherwise."

Just before the 2012 Games began, the Transplant Games of America announced it would plan games in 2014 and 2016, that it was entertaining bids from more than twelve cities across the country, and that it was expected that more cities would follow.

That announcement has come to fruition with the 2014 Games held in Houston, the 2016 Games in Cleveland, the 2018 Games in Salt Lake City, and the 2020 Games set to take place in Meadowlands, New Jersey.

Prior to his transplant, Fred says he had never heard of the Transplant Games. But as he recovered, the games would prove to be a source of motivation and inspiration for him. Fred would experience firsthand the impact of the games, as well as the impact they've had on thousands of transplant recipients, living donors, donor families, and others.

18

"Rise Like a Phoenix…"

"I'm sure there will be people able to bring tears to my eyes, because if I thought I had it bad, there's always someone in worse shape. I use the analogy of a phoenix rising from the ashes. That's the celebration we're going to have this weekend. There's going to be hundreds of phoenixes that rise, and we're going to fly together and celebrate life."

–Fred Nelis

Gordon closed out 2015 in the hospital.

He had been doing well for eighteen months and his FEV1 had been at 100 percent for more than a year. In that span of time, it seemed he had drunk from the Fountain of Youth.

He had come a long way since staring at death's door in June 2014. From a severely limited life of sitting immobile and trying to catch his breath, he was now doing all of the things he loved: biking, kayaking, sailing, traveling. He and Nancy had put on a lot of miles in the past year and half.

He had also spent the past months trying to convince his caregivers that a six-week trip to New Zealand was just what he needed to continue on that upward trajectory.

"The transplant went pretty smoothly, and he did incredibly well for a period of time," said Dr. Girgis. "But we did struggle with him wanting to do his own thing," he added. "He was pretty non-compliant to say the least; stubborn, he felt he knew his body better than others did."

According to Nancy and other friends, he was not being compliant with his medications and was not doing his prescribed pulmonary exercises.

"He couldn't, or wouldn't do them," Nancy recalled.

In December, Gordon was scheduled for a bronchoscopy with biopsy, a much more invasive procedure than Fred's heart biopsies, in which a tube is inserted through the windpipe into the lung, so that tissue samples can be extracted. There was concern that he might be suffering rejection as his FEV1 had dropped to 78 percent in his latest exam.

The biopsy revealed that he was indeed suffering an acute rejection crisis, and he was admitted to the hospital immediately, where an IV delivered 1,000 milligrams of Prednisone daily—ten times the amount that Fred had been prescribed during his mild rejection episode.

Gordon told Fred afterward that during the treatment every nerve in his body had been alive and throbbing. He said that he felt so on edge that it seemed as if his eyes were popping out of his head.

"I think the seriousness of rejection scared him enough to consent to treatment and be compliant with the additional breathing therapy," Fred recalled.

Even so, Gordon remained a man on the move, and if he was running from his hopeless past and from the pain and discomfort of his present treatment, he was also running toward something.

"To have something to look forward to is quite possibly the most important thing in life," he told Fred and Jean at a dinner in early 2016, shortly after his hospitalization. "With Nancy I have a future now."

What the couple had been planning and looking forward to for months was about to come to fruition. They would set off on a six-week excursion to New Zealand in February. Gordon had long had a special affinity for the people of New Zealand. He admired the Kiwis' love of sport, the outdoors, and travel. Despite the nation's relatively small population, it seemed that no matter where you ventured in the world, you would inevitably happen upon a New Zealander. He also enjoyed their friendliness and the "mate" culture that cherished the bonds of friendship.

In early February, the couple flew to San Diego, visited Nancy's parents again, and then drove to Los Angeles, where they boarded a flight to Auckland. After a brief stay with Fred's sister-in-law Megan Nelis's family and a bit of traveling on the North Island, they flew to Christchurch, where they picked up a camper complete with bathroom, kitchen, grill, and all of the other amenities they would need for an extended sojourn around the South Island.

The spine of the South Island is composed of the Southern Alps, towering peaks that often rise to 10,000 feet or more. On the east side lies the Canterbury Plain, while the west is a dramatic maze of rugged coastlines and glaciers. The dramatic setting has been the production location for a number of films in recent years, including the *Lord of the Rings* trilogy.

Throughout their journey, the couple went where their interests led them—covering long distances some days and traveling very little on others. Each night they would pull the camper over and park alongside the ocean, preparing a meal together they would share under the stars. There was no need of a campground, although they made the concession of stopping into one every so often for a shower. Gordon did the driving, and Nancy said that "he did very well, despite all of the mountains and curves and driving on the left side of the road."

Nancy's most vivid memory of the trip comes from the North Island, where Gordon and Nancy visited the famous Hot Water Beach on the east coast of the Coromandel Peninsula. Surrounded by volcanos, the beach sits atop geothermal fissures through which volcanic springs seep up into the sand, creating an instant, private spa for beachgoers.

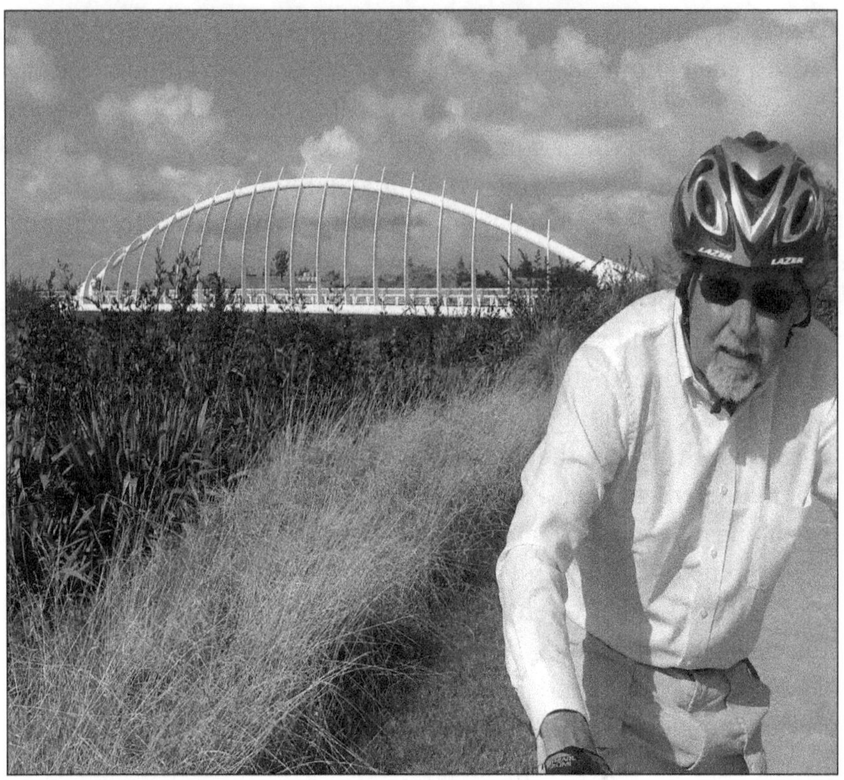

Gordon in New Zealand biking

They arrived at a nearby campground in the evening and spoke to several campers who informed them that the hot springs are dependent on the tide, and that they'd better get there early the next day to carve out space on the beach. Gordon turned to Nancy and said, "The hell with it, why wait twelve hours to share the beach with a cast of thousands? Let's go now."

"So we got on our bikes and there was not a soul on the beach," Nancy said. "We had the whole beach to ourselves. We took off our suits, plopped down in the sand, and watched the Southern Cross. After that trip, I had a hard time with trips that had an itinerary. I loved having the freedom of going where you wanted to."

The couple put close to 3,000 miles on their camper throughout the six-week trip. Upon their return to the US, however, Nancy noticed a change in Gordon.

"I was worried because of his health," she said.

She was not the only one to note a change.

"After Gordon went through treatment for rejection in December I think he realized his frailty," Fred recalled. "He assured me that he learned his lesson and made assurances to the clinic about his compliance with daily medicine dosages."

"When he got back, even though he was mentally invigorated, I could see a significant downdraft in his energy levels," he added.

Since their successful surgeries, Fred and Gordon had made it a point to get together on a regular basis—at least once a month. Throughout the spring and summer of 2016, Fred notes they didn't see each other as often.

"He came back sick and laid low for a little while," Fred said. "I think he came back more sober to the reality that he had lit the candle at both ends."

"When Gordon came back from New Zealand, his lung function was quite a bit lower," Dr. Girgis noted. His FEV1 had yet to return to the 100 percent he had enjoyed for more than a year.

In February, as Jean nervously fretted, Fred participated in his first US Masters swim meet since the transplant. Fred's performance at Grand Haven High School showed that he had a long way to go.

"I was disappointed," Fred recalled. "Jean was there and I had friends there. Here I was in the middle of people who knew me and my swimming accomplishments and I was brought back to reality. It was very humbling."

"It's not where you want to be after forty-five years of competitive swimming," he added. "No matter what I knew or how I trained, it was a struggle and a painful one at that."

Fred admits nerves played a part. After his performance, he continued to train, seeking answers in preparation for his next challenge—The Transplant Games of America, which would take place in Cleveland, June 10–15, only four months after Grand Haven.

For a normal heart transplant patient, there would be nothing embarrassing about the times Fred swam in Grand Haven. In fact, they were not far off the times that some of his Transplant Games of America competitors would swim later that summer. But Fred held himself to a different standard. At the very least, the experience provided him a baseline from which to mark his improvement. He knew he had a number of physical, technical and mental challenges to overcome in the next 120 days of preparation.

Physically, he had some valid excuses for his performance. Often, heart transplant patients begin recovery with a condition called a "stiff heart," which may take months or even years to improve. This occurs because the nerve bundle attached to a normal heart is severed with transplantation. The only method of signaling the heart that it is "show time," or time to pump faster, comes from the adrenal glands rather than electrical stimulation from the brain. Whereas a signal from the brain would start the heart pounding immediately, there is a lag in the time necessary for the body to produce adrenaline. Long, slow warmups are crucial to jumpstarting this process. For Fred that meant almost twenty minutes or 1,000 yards of warmup before things started working smoothly.

There were other physical issues in addition to the stiff heart. During his LVAD surgery he had suffered a collapsed lung and damage to the phrenic nerve that controls the left diaphragm. Twenty months post-surgery, the nerve damage had yet to completely heal.

Fred also suffered from thoracic outlet syndrome in his left arm, a condition in which blood vessels and nerves in the space between the collarbone and ribs are compressed as in the case of carpal tunnel in the wrist. The condition causes pain and numbness in the shoulder, arm, and fingers.

"The thoracic outlet syndrome lasted throughout and beyond Cleveland," Fred said. "The blood supply doesn't get to the arm muscle. Even if your heart is pumping like a racehorse, there is nothing in there but lactic acid. There are operations they can do," he added. "But I am not going in for another operation."

From a technical standpoint, Fred needed to develop a strategy to deal with the stiff heart that would allow sufficient warm-up without burning him out prior to the race, and sufficient warm-down without tiring him for his next race.

Over the next few months, Fred began to show slight improvement in his quest to win a medal in Cleveland. He studied his workout routines and found that shorter lengths with more rest proved more profitable than longer workouts with short rest.

"I write down all of my workouts," Fred recalled. "During this time, I made continual improvements, which gave me some improved confidence, but I still didn't have my usual stamina."

Fred will tell you that swimming is every bit as much a thinking sport as golf or chess. The slightest change of the placement of the hand or the head might result in the hundredth of a second that means the difference between gold and silver.

"I just wasn't smart enough in Grand Haven," he reflected. "I thought I could just get out there and bang it out. It's a learning process."

In addition to the thinking part, there is a psychological component at work in the mind of every competitor. For Fred, that meant once again finding the confidence that would give him the winning edge.

"I could see progress, but the hardest thing for me to do was to learn how to race again," he said. "Once you lose that edge, you are just swimming, not racing. That's what I was doing at the time. I didn't have the confidence.

"My resolve was tested," Fred said. "The seasoned competitor in me said, 'Just go out there and do the best you can, and accept the congratulations for doing way less than you're used to being able to do,'" he added. "I was just praying this wasn't the best I'd ever be able to do."

THE DIRTY DUDES and Dusty Dames enjoyed their first four-wheeling weekend of 2016 in April. It was a cold one and there was still snow on the ground. But the outing gave Fred the opportunity to unveil his latest T-shirt, gray this time, emblazoned with the slogan "Rise like a phoenix, soar like an eagle," and complete with a depiction of the mythical bird.

According to Greek mythology, the 500-year-old phoenix cyclically obtains new life by rising from the ashes of its predecessor. Some sources portray the phoenix dying in a fiery shower of flames, while others claim that the legendary bird dies and simply decomposes before being born again.

Despite the high-flying slogans and corresponding T-shirts, Fred was business as usual as he continued to prepare for the next milestone in his recovery. Prior to his transplant, Fred says that he did not know competitions such as the Transplant Games existed. As a new transplant recipient, he had made it his goal to begin training as soon as possible after transplant.

In the weeks leading up to the event, Fred and Jean decided they would go to Cleveland alone. Although the event was within easy driving distance of family and friends, who would have jumped at the opportunity to cheer Fred on, he was haunted by his performance in Grand Haven and chose to keep a low profile in case things went the way they had in February.

Prior to leaving for the Games, he was interviewed by several local TV stations. He told WXMI TV-17 reporter Erica Francis that he thought his T-shirt best summed up his approach to what would take place over the coming days in Cleveland.

"I'm sure there will be people able to bring tears to my eyes, because if I thought I had it bad, there's always someone in worse shape," Fred said. "I use the analogy of a phoenix rising from the ashes. That's the celebration we're going to have this weekend. There's going to be hundreds of phoenixes that rise, and we're going to fly together and celebrate life. Out of the ashes you have a second chance and that second chance brings you the opportunity to soar like an eagle," he added.

Fred also says he felt added pressure because he was not only racing for himself, but for an anonymous 32-year-old organ donor as well.

"This is the first time I'm going to race for the two of us," Nelis told *Health Beat* in an interview at the Games. "I've trained and gotten stronger, but this is the first time I'm going to race with my donor and me."

FRED ARRIVED IN Cleveland with some apprehension, but also with his typical determination. Although he had spoken to Holly Werlein and others about previous games, it was a whole new experience, and quite distinct from a typical swim meet.

When Fred looked around at the other competitors, he saw men and women, boys and girls, young and old, all shapes and sizes. Many had been competitive athletes like Fred and had great physiques. Many bore scars on their abdomens, chests, backs, and torsos. Many competed with the name of their donor or the date of their transplant written onto their skin, and almost to the person, they had terrific smiles on their faces.

But the biggest impact for Fred and Jean occurred before Fred even had a chance to dip a toe in the water. Saturday night, in the opening ceremonies of the Transplant Games, organizers honored donors and families of donors.

"It was so emotional," Jean said. "The athletes all come in by their states, and then the living donors and donor families come in. And they get more applause than the athletes."

That experience put everything in perspective for Fred and enabled him to take his mark the next day with a clear mind and a sense of purpose.

Frequently, "brushing my teeth, washing my face, standing at the mirror—I look at the scars that are on my chest," Fred told *Health Beat*. "And I know they're there because someone else gave me another chance. Someone who didn't know me.

"I just sit there and get chills thinking about it," he said. "It happens every single day. The newness, the freshness, it hasn't worn off. It's there every time I look at my chest. There's somebody else inside of me."

Health Beat's Shawn Foucher was on hand the next day to document Fred's return to competitive racing.

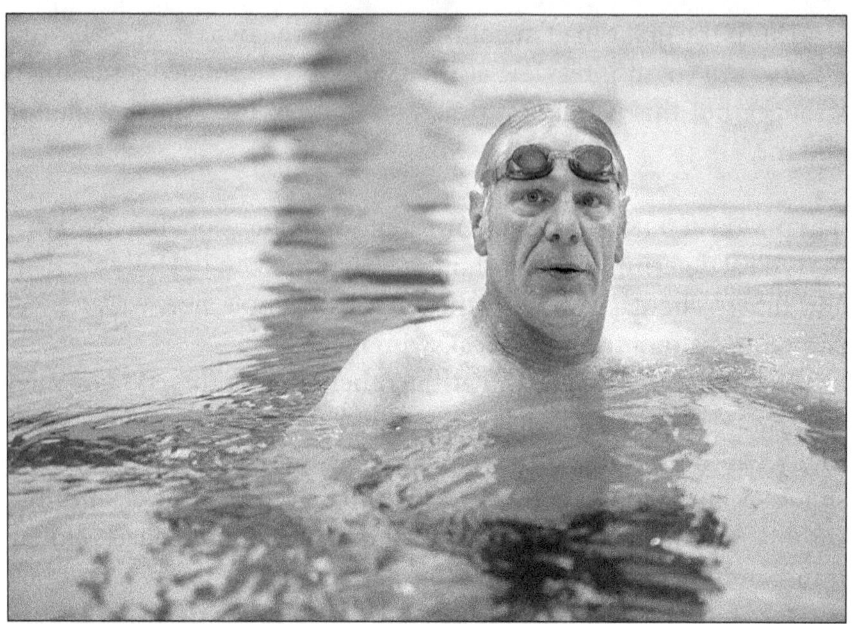

Warming up prior to the Transplant Games in Cleveland

On the first day of competition, as he toed the mark for the 50-yard backstroke, he had butterflies and felt apprehensive.

For a moment.

'It was pretty much gone after that 50-yard backstroke. That would have been my weakest race—but I set a tone for the other races,' Fred said.

About that tone.

The 50-yard backstroke, first place. The 100-yard freestyle, first place. The 50-yard butterfly, first place. The 50-yard freestyle, first place.

At that point, it was as if a weight had been lifted from Fred's shoulders. For the rest of the weekend, it was all about celebrating with his teammates and Jean, expressing his gratitude and enjoying the camaraderie of his fellow competitors.

"IT'S ABOUT GIVING PEOPLE
THEIR LIVES BACK"

"Fred is a poster child for transplants," said his cardiologist, Dr. Mike Dickinson. "The Transplant Games are done to raise community awareness and celebrate the gift of life so the world can see that a transplant is not just about keeping people alive in a hospital or nursing home—it's about giving people their lives back."

BILL KLAHN, A veteran swimmer of many Transplant Games, approached Fred on Sunday after noticing his impressive debut.

"You know," he told Fred, "we're going to go to the World Games next year in Spain, and we'd really like to have you swim. I think we might be able to medal in the team relays."

Fred's new goal emerged: the 21st World Transplant Games in Malaga, located on Spain's Costa del Sol, in summer 2017.

"I think it might make a nice family vacation this time around," Fred said with a smile and a new reason to begin training.

19

Whence Cometh My Help?

"I had never been terribly prayerful. But I had this perception: It's not about petition, it's about reception. Our tiny little minds can't even communicate what we need."

—FRED NELIS

DESPITE THE SURFACE DIFFERENCES in personality, beliefs, circumstance, and adherence to doctors' orders, when you watch Fred and Gordon with people or speak to them for any length of time, some commonalities emerge.

Both men are highly social and good at bringing out the best in other people. They excel at brightening the lives of others. Both feel immense sorrow for the family of their organ donor, and extreme gratitude for the second chance at life they have been given. Both are ready and eager to seize that opportunity, hoist it, and drain it to the dregs.

Both men relish the physical rebirth that is allowing them to do things that were impossible just a few short years and even months ago. Both still grapple with the profound connection that unites them in body, spirit, and mind.

"Gordon and I have a very close and unique bond because we share something that not even brothers share," Fred says, trying to put his concepts into words.

"I have a hard time comprehending it," Gordon says.

"It's a bond that's hard to describe. I'm not sure I have the linguistic skill to do so," Fred says, giving up for the time being, though it will not be the last time he wrestles with what it means to be conjoined with Gordon.

It also becomes clear that both Fred and Gordon are capable of transcendent spiritual, emotional, and psychological experiences. Fred chooses to characterize his experiences within the spiritual context of his Catholic faith. Gordon, on the other hand, embraces transcendent experience as part of a philosophical materialism that operates without need of an all-powerful, sentient deity and beyond the confines of traditional, organized religion.

Fred's faith and the practice of his religion trace back to his earliest upbringing and the influence of his parents. But his is not a superficial religious practice carried on solely for the sake of tradition. Throughout his life, he has been drawn in a profound, spiritual way to examples of sacrifice, compassion, duty, and devotion.

Fred has mentioned his lifelong fascination with the symbolism of the Sacred Heart of Jesus, a devotion that is especially concerned with the longsuffering love and compassion of the heart of Christ toward humanity.

He is also intrigued by the concept of the Trinity and the Pentecost, which celebrates the descent of the Holy Spirit on the disciples of Jesus after His ascension.

"The promise of the Pentecost is that you will never be left alone," Fred explains. "The power of the Holy Spirit fell on all of those who were present.

"The Spirit told them, 'What I have done is nothing compared to the miracles you will perform in the name of the Father.' And you develop such power through faith in the reconciliation and the gift of the Spirit," he adds. "In my journey, I have felt that Spirit in more than one situation."

Never more strongly or profoundly than on the date of his idio-pathic cardiomyopathy diagnosis. On the dark night of January 7, 1994 at 8:00 p.m.—Fred remembers the exact date and time—he stood alone at a window, facing north, on the top floor of Holland Hospital.

"I felt this calm, this whisper, this inclination. I don't know how to explain. It was more of a sense of 'Ask Me,'" he recounts.

It was the first time he'd had such a premonition, encounter—call it what you will—and he admits to feeling more than a little "shell-shocked" from his experiences of the day. But he continued standing, and as the feeling started to dissipate, he felt a tap on the shoulder and a more insistent and specific question: "What is it that you would have?"

Aware how this might sound to a nonbeliever, Fred is, nonethe-less, convinced that this was the Holy Spirit calling out to him, and concedes that, under the circumstances, the first thing a normal per-son would ask for would be the restoration of health. But he recalled Solomon's response to God's question: "What is it that you would have from me? Power, glory, money?" Solomon, instead, asked for wisdom, and through that gift was able to obtain the rest.

"I wasn't trying to outsmart God," Fred said. "But I thought of Solomon and I asked for something different. I asked for acceptance and not having anger about my situation.

"At that point I had one of those personal, deeply mystical experi-ences, like fairy dust sprinkling down on my head. I had this sudden rush of warmth and nerve activity, a tingling, kind of prickly, you know how the sun warms you from head to toe? I still don't have the words, but it was a kind of internal and external glow that filled me," he said.

Fred says that night was the beginning of a profound shift that changed his understanding of and relationship with God.

"Many people try to be prayerful," he said. "I had never been ter-ribly prayerful. But I had this perception: It's not about petition, it's about reception. Our tiny little minds can't even communicate what we need.

"I wanted to have an acceptance of whatever I was in for, and not to blame anything or anyone for what I had and instead look at it as an opportunity for growth," he said. "I didn't want to use anger as an escape, despite my competitive nature."

That receptivity and the feelings of acceptance and gratitude have stayed with him for two plus decades and allowed him a measure of peace.

"I had this perception that this gift I got in 1994 was going to sustain me," Fred said. "The night I was going to have my transplant I was absolutely relaxed and at peace. I felt comfortable with my decision, tried to reassure the family, and was very positive. I just felt I was being held in a bubble of comfort."

Fred admits there was a moment when he did give in to his anger. "The only time I ever got angry between that point and after the transplant was when I had issues with my eyesight," he said. "But that wasn't directed to the Almighty, but toward the humanity that took care of me."

But even that negative experience turned into a positive.

"My internist sent me to a new cardiologist, Mike Dickinson," he said. "The first thing he did was adjust the meds, and I mentally and physically felt better. For me that burst of anger did have positive results."

Gordon has a similar appreciation of silver linings. Looking back on his life, Gordon admits that he has had both extremely good and extremely bad fortune. And many things in his life that he initially thought of as negatives turned into positives:

"The shooting in Milwaukee was a negative that turned into a positive because there were no long-term ramifications," he said. "I got to learn about mortality at an early age and that was the best knowledge I ever had."

But Gordon took a different path than Fred to come to these hard-won conclusions.

"Gordon had a lot of anger inside of him that didn't come out very often but that was bubbling just below the surface," said ex-wife

Beverly Fogarty. "He felt like the odd duck during his Christian Reformed upbringing, and was a confirmed atheist."

Although he joined the Unitarian Church in Ludington during his marriage to Beverly, he did so mainly to widen his social circle. According to Beverly, he didn't go to church very often because he didn't like hymns, and he was very irreverent.

"He loves Christmas, but the secular version," she said. "He was always very derogatory about Christians in general. I guess he thought they were always too judgmental."

"I do have a god and it is called DNA," Gordon says. "God is here forever; DNA is here forever; it makes us and we are an exact copy of what it wants us to be. We are an electrochemical process, and we have what we call 'consciousness' because we have the ability to remember the past."

However, Gordon maintains respect for his Transplant Brother's beliefs.

"Fred is not your average Christian—not in the same way as the sect I was brought up in," Gordon says. "They are rabidly Christian. I had no idea about Fred's religious persuasion until someone told me."

"Mine was a merciful and loving God compared to Gordon's," Fred replies.

Gordon's parents were charter members of a Christian Reformed Church in Grand Rapids, where his father served as an elder. Following the influx of Dutch emigration that began in the mid-nineteenth century, West Michigan became a bastion of Calvinist scholarship and worship.

Things have changed in the decades since, but in the 1950s and '60s when Gordon was growing up, many West Michigan children of religious families were required to spend their Sabbath in quiet contemplation of their spiritual state. Neighbors who broke the Sabbath by mowing their lawn, washing their car, playing loud music, or, heaven forbid, drinking a beer on their porch, were regarded with heretical wonder. These children were also often forbidden to attend dances or to watch movies or television.

Gordon recalled, "In the Church, I couldn't go to dances or movies. Outside that world, I got high on being alive.

"What used to get me was being at the summer house at Lake Michigan on a beautiful Sunday," he said. "We'd have to sit inside and reflect on our sinfulness. It was so bizarre.

"And the funerals, you know what's so funny about the funerals? They never mentioned the person," he added. "What are we doing here? I could never buy any of it."

"I recall Gordon telling my parents at one point that he wasn't going to church anymore," Gordon's sister Margo recalled. "My dad said that as long as you live at home, you are going with us."

Jean Nelis grew up in the Reformed Church of America, but her parents were more open-minded and accepting than Gordon's.

"I'm Catholic," Jean reminds us, converting when the girls were young. "My sister is Unitarian, one brother has no church affiliation, and the other brother is Reformed and his wife is a minister. My parents always accepted the differences in our beliefs."

Gordon was a big fan of Jean's father, Harold Vande Bunte Jr., who passed away in 2012 at the age of 86. In fact, Jean's father was the first Vande Bunte to befriend Gordon, getting to know him when Gordon serviced the Xerox machines in the pharmacies he owned and operated for many years in downtown Holland and Zeeland. He would later introduce Gordon to his son, John, a yacht designer, when he learned of Gordon's love of sailing.

"John and Jean's father was so accepting and so free with his smiles and positive comments," Gordon recalled. "Even if he didn't know you and you showed up at their cottage on Bills Lake, if John said you were a friend, you were fine."

Jean married a man whose personal mission in life, in some ways, resembles that of her father. Fred may not be quite as easygoing as Harold Vande Bunte, but when asked to describe an accomplishment that makes a day complete, Fred responds with the following:

"The thing I'd like to do if I could do it every day is bump into someone who wasn't feeling red hot and at least harass them enough to make them smile just a little bit," he said. "That would be the perfect day—to make someone feel better."

"Fred is kind-hearted," says longtime friend Dave Siegers, a former member of the Dutch Masters swim club. "He believes that God has meaning and purpose in his life, and he does what he can to have a positive impact on people."

After all that Fred and his family have been through, it may come as no surprise that he finds a special affinity and inspiration in the trials and tribulations of Job.

"Even after Job lost everything, he never cursed God," says Fred. "The devil would plant the seeds with his friends and in Job's mind, telling him, 'There is no reason not to curse God—you are being punished for things that are not your fault.' Despite all of the things that happened, he never lost his faith.

"Whatever could happen to that guy did," Fred adds. "And yet at the end he is restored to his fullness."

Fred also has expectations of an afterlife.

"If we read the Scriptures, there is this anticipation of a promise of life in which the tears will be wiped away and the brokenness will be mended," he says. "It is a harmony we have escaped here. I don't have any contemplation of what that would be—a level of fullness or completeness in which we are one with God, a blissful existence, not necessarily in a corporal sense, but perhaps in a spiritual sense."

Gordon's sister Margo continues to worry about the condition of her brother's immortal soul.

"We have a burden for Gordon's soul," she said, adding that the last time she visited him in the hospital, she asked him if he had an assurance of heaven. "That's very important to me. I want to know where I'm going when I die."

Gordon's concerns are more grounded to the earth.

"As for what happens after, when that electrochemical process stops, we are, for all practical purposes done, and there is nothing left afterwards except our memory and our legacy," he says. "I'm 99…I'm 100 percent sure of that."

Both Jean and Nancy pay less heed to doctrine, ignore some of Gordon's bluster, and consider him to be a very spiritual person—just in a different way than Fred.

"Gordon is anti-religion but is still very spiritual," Jean says. "Look at Fred and Gordon. They are a miracle. If you can't see that, you are ignoring the facts.

"To me, the world is a miracle. It doesn't matter if it is evolution or God's hand in evolution," she adds. "Gord isn't against accepting that. He is just against people telling him what to believe.

"Gordon is more of a spiritual person," agrees Nancy. "He has a real love for animals and plants, almost to the degree of being like a religion."

Part of Gordon's love for the country and people of New Zealand, apart from visiting his old friends, the Siewerts, has to do with the traditional Maori outlook and their relation to their natural surroundings—a oneness and an existential and familial link they share with all living creatures, the forest, the land, and the sea.

In fact, as Gordon and Nancy battled Gordon's physicians for approval of their grand New Zealand adventure in early 2016, Gordon repeatedly waxed ecstatic about the New Zealand Parliament's 2015 Animal Welfare Amendment legislation. This law, among many other requirements, formally recognized animals as sentient beings, banned their use in cosmetic testing, required animal owners to attend properly to their welfare, and established a National Animal Welfare Advisory Committee and a National Animal Ethics Advisory Committee.

"That's why I'm happy to go to New Zealand," Gordon said before he and Nancy set out on their trip. "They have just voted to pass a law on the sanctity of animals. I am delighted that a national government has taken such steps, and even though I bluster about the Christians, I tolerate them as well.

"Studying biology and the chemistry of life and the fact that our brains are so typical of mammalians, why do we have eternal life and the orangutan that is 99 percent genetically similar to us doesn't?" he asked rhetoricall

20

A Bittersweet Anniversary

"I built up that ledge with wheelbarrow after wheelbarrow of sand, pushed straight up the hill. I was so powerful back then, I was like a machine."

—Gordon Veldman

FRED, JEAN, AND MY WIFE and I drove up to Pentwater to spend time with Gordon and Nancy on June 17, 2017—the day prior to the three-year anniversary of Fred and Gordon's transplant surgery.

It was a glorious June day in Michigan—nothing but clear blue sky and the hint of a cool breeze blowing off Pentwater Lake as we pulled into town. We partially circumnavigated the lake that lies at the heart of the village after we missed the steep and circuitous turnoff that snakes its way up to Gordon's lair, high atop a wooded hillside overlooking the lake.

Pentwater is a sleepy little hamlet of less than 1,000 souls in winter. Its population swells in the summer as a literal cottage industry of tourists, boutique and bed-and-breakfast owners, arts-and-crafts sellers, sailors, retirees, Chicagoans, and other summer people flock to its sparkling shoreline.

I had visited Gordon in the hospital in April and, at that time, it had been some months since I'd seen him in person. Nancy was sitting next to the bed when I walked in, helping him to reach something on his nightstand—a glass of water perhaps. My reaction to seeing him was, no doubt, reminiscent of something he said to me when I interviewed him the first time:

"I could see my mortality reflected in the eyes of my friends," he said, when he described his lowest ebb prior to being listed for a transplant.

Gone was the bluff and blustery practical joker, the mischievous adventurer, the restless and searching spirit, the charming raconteur. In its place was the look of a tired, resigned, and defeated man, for whom speech and breath were immense efforts.

I had spoken to him several times by telephone in the intervening two months, however, and he sounded much stronger than he had appeared on that April day.

Fred, however, had spoken with him on the phone just the previous day. He told us on the drive up that we should prepare ourselves to be surprised again at Gordon's condition.

"He is disappointed things are going this way again," Fred said. "I think he is very angry with his physical state."

I practiced a look of neutrality in the rearview mirror as we made our way past Muskegon on US 31. At first glance, it seemed unnecessary.

Gordon appeared much more hale and hearty than he had in April. There was color in his cheeks, a rosy glow, not the cyanosis associated with low oxygen levels in the red blood cells or problems circulating oxygenated blood that had plagued him in previous times.

"A gigantic pain in the ass is what I've created here," he responded to my enthusiastic commentary as I took in the breadth and depth of his property's idiosyncrasies.

Gordon's home and property have been described as "like something from *The Hobbit*." Perhaps a perpetually restless and curious

6'4" hobbit. My impression was that of an abode that evolved and grew directly from the whims of its handy, though largely self-taught, proprietor.

High on a hill overlooking Pentwater Lake, the wooden house with its giant steel deck that once featured a rope swing arching out into the void looks almost hand-carved, hewn and forged out of the surrounding woods and environment. In its wake lie a scattering of other rough-hewn structures—a woodworking shop and a shed that houses the wood-burning, smoke-spewing furnace, the source of heat for the whole property. Giant koi mark time in an almost-infinity pond, blissfully ignorant of the marvelous view of the lake. Carved wooden hands and a wooden nose sprout whimsically from a large tree near the garage. Inside the house, a jumble of remarkable items comprises a décor apropos of no identifiable school outside of the "Gordwardian Way," from Buddhist artifacts to antique model cars, homemade wood furniture, and colorful glass sculptures hanging from an acrylic skylight.

"It used to be a straight hillside over there," he points out. "Now with the ledge I built it's hard to tell."

"I built up that ledge with wheelbarrow after wheelbarrow of sand, pushed straight up the hill," he adds. "I was so powerful back then, I was like a machine."

My wife and I continue to compliment him on the property. I, with the real enthusiasm of one who has long tired of the charms of our cookie-cutter, suburban bi-level, and she, more likely out of admiration for the sheer audacity of the place.

Gordon describes himself as "an amateur woodworker, turned into a steelworker." It turns out that he designed the steel deck himself to contain a reinforced cross piece and bridge truss. He initiated the project at the Pentwater Artisan Learning Center, where he teaches welding on a volunteer basis.

"As always, they said, 'Let's see the plans' and then rolled their eyes when I pointed at my head and said they were up here," Gordon said.

"Sure enough, they thought, 'There goes another boondoggle by that guy we have watched go off on so many tangents,'" he said. "I will tell you something though. If you are the only one on a project, there doesn't need to be anything on paper because you don't have to pass information. I corrected the situation as I went along.

"Over the winter, I welded it all up. Because the design was so fluid in my mind I was able to come up against situations and correct them as I went. For example, this cross piece—when I supported it like it was supposed to be supported, I jumped on it and bent it, so I thought I can't have that, so I put the bridge strut beneath it."

Improvising one's way through life is a central tenet of the Gordwardian Way, I had been informed by his closest friends.

We sit outside soaking in the sun and talking, enjoying visits from several squirrels, a squadron of ruby-throated humming-birds sipping nectar, and the eventual arrival of a bald eagle, whose thick-limbed nest the size of a Volkswagen perches in a tree on the property. Gordon tells us more about the life he has carved out in this little neck of the woods, in the only county in Michigan without a traffic light.

"I have a group I get together with every Tuesday night. They are locals—nice description of rednecks," he says. "We just drink a beer around the campfire. Three quarters of them have never been in an airplane.

"There's a lot of people who can't afford to have their arm set if they broke it," he continued. "I have had contact with every department of the hospital, many times and often. It just boggles my mind the difference between health insurance and no health insurance. It is so bizarre to have this situation."

As the sun passes overhead and shadows lengthen, however, it becomes apparent that Gordon is tiring. Getting up to use the restroom requires significant effort, and after his third trip inside he has to rest on the sofa before coming out to the deck to rejoin us.

"I'm on Lasix, my ankles are retaining water, I have to pee every half hour," he says with just a trace of bitterness. "I have all I can do to walk out of my house to walk to my walker.

"Three years ago tomorrow," he muses. "You know what, Jean, it's almost a bittersweet moment for me now. I realize what has come and gone and I just keep hoping there will be a little bit bigger window to crawl through to live in. But there is no reserve anymore.

"They wanted me to continue the treatment for Alpha-1 deficiency after transplant, but it is such an invasive and expensive affair and I don't trust the company to give me anything of remote quality," he says. "It was eleven thousand dollars a month. I chose not to. There may have been mistakes made in how I set up my life post-transplant. The shoulda coulda wouldas…

"They have me on a machine at night," he adds. "And I really question that because my thought is my lungs should be the ones to work. Why let a machine force them to work? I really have to question that."

We get up finally to drive to a late lunch. Fred suggests that Gordon bring an oxygen tank and his walker. I offer to carry both. Gordon will have nothing to do with either. It takes us an eternity to walk out to Fred and Jean's car.

Our destination is the Pentwater Yacht Club. The parking lot is full and the nearest parking space is three blocks away. There is no way Gordon will be able to walk that distance, so the decision is made to head to a place in Hart, about fifteen minutes away, famous for its fried chicken.

Jean pulls the car up close to the entrance for Gordon, but he insists that we all enter rather than wait for him to make the arduous climb out of the back seat and into the restaurant. Fred and Jean and my wife, Ilsy, and I enter the restaurant while Nancy remains with Gordon.

We have time to find a table and visit the restroom to wash our hands. As I make my way back to the table, Gordon is just getting seated.

Things are obviously worse than they appeared upon our arrival.

Gordon is putting on a brave front for our benefit and talks about having my whole family out for a visit in July when we return from Spain. I heartily agree, knowing that my twelve- and ten-year-olds would love hanging out with him, exploring his house, and goofing around in his yard. Kids love Gordon.

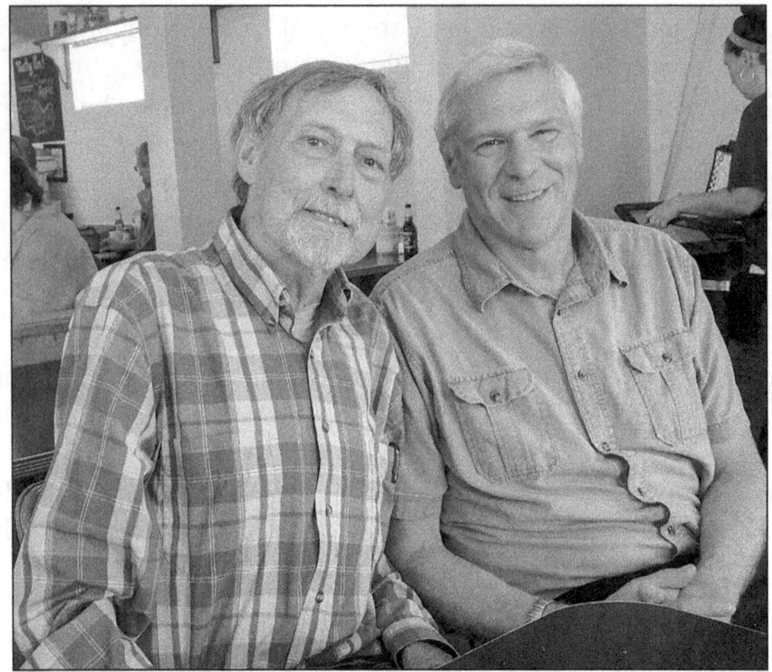

Last pic of transplant brothers together

The daughter of a former girlfriend of Gordon's had told me that she prayed he would become her stepfather, unfortunately to no avail.

I dig into my fried chicken platter with relish. They are correct. The place has great fried chicken, something I love but rarely get the chance to eat. Jean, Nancy, and my wife also eat with gusto. The food is really good. Fred eats carefully. I'm not sure how much of this is due to him being a picky eater and how much is due to the care with which he maintains his diet.

Fred is the antithesis of Gordon when it comes to following his doctor's wishes. There is no railing against the system, no complaints or non-compliance. Fred is intelligent and will investigate the best care available, bouncing questions off his daughter Jami, a nurse, and his niece, Emily, a cardiologist. But once he has committed, he is 100 percent committed as he is in all areas of his life. Today he eats carefully, nourished with the knowledge and gratitude that he has been given another chance.

At one point, I feel that I catch a meaningful glance from Gordon. It occurs just after we agree to visit in July. He starts to say something, is interrupted by the flow of conversation, and never gets a chance to get back to what he wanted to say.

Gordon's plate is hardly touched. We finish, the talk winds down, and my wife takes yet another photograph of Fred and Gordon together before we head home.

It turns out to be the last photograph ever taken of the Transplant Brothers together.

21

Two Journeys:
Malaga, Andalucía, Spain,
and Grand Rapids, Michigan

"Nancy, I don't know how long I'm going to live."

—Gordon Veldman

"We are all living on borrowed time, but for a transplant recipient that realization is even more concentrated."

—Fred Nelis

AS WAS MENTIONED in an earlier chapter, Nancy's memory of New Zealand's Hot Water Beach on the east coast of the North Island's Coromandel Peninsula is one of the most vivid of her travels there with Gordon.

But it isn't just the couple's impromptu, midnight bicycle trip to reach the volcanic springs on the beach that sticks in her mind. She also recalls a conversation they shared while they luxuriated together under the stars.

As they sat there enjoying the moment, Gordon turned to her and said, *"Nancy, I don't know how long I'm going to live."*

"He felt like he was on borrowed time," she said. "But I always pooh-poohed it, saying there are people who live for twenty years with transplants."

Sometime in the second week of June 2017, about a week before Fred, Jean, and my wife and I visited them, Gordon turned to Nancy one morning and said, "Nancy, this feels different in my chest."

"He knew what rejection felt like," she said. "He had been down that road before. But it was like he knew something and didn't want to upset me."

It had been a rough late winter and spring for the couple.

A month-long trip to Key West to visit old friends in February had started pleasantly enough, but Gordon picked up a cold there and could not shake it when they returned to Michigan. By April both Nancy and Gordon were sick. Nancy eventually recovered from her cold, but Gordon's lingered, turning to pneumonia.

After a visit to the ER, Gordon was admitted to the hospital for 18 days. While undergoing treatment, a breathing tube was required. Nancy spent much of the next 18 days with him and noted that his arterial blood gasses were double the normal amount. It got to the point where he didn't know what he was doing, at times becoming violent, lashing out, and one time pushing Nancy as she tried to help him.

I visited Gordon at the tail end of this hospital stay, and like others, was shocked at the change in his appearance.

Upon discharge, to avoid further hospitalization for pulmonary rehabilitation, Nancy says that Gordon promised to abide by all rules, take his meds, wear his BPAP (Bilevel Positive Airway Pressure) machine at night, and do his own rehab at home.

"I stayed with him the first week," she said. "He was good about everything that week, but after that he was not being compliant. He was good for about 10 days and then started going downhill."

Gordon was seen by pulmonologist Ryan Hadley, MD, on June 11, and Nancy reports he was told, "There is no reason you can't lead a normal life. I'd like to see you on your bike and getting exercise."

As they were leaving the clinic, Gordon was given a big hug by JaNae, one of the nurses who had cared for him post-transplant.

"He told me that he took that as a final hug," Nancy recalled. "I didn't know what to think. He was such a conspiracy theorist."

However, he began using oxygen tanks more regularly, and Nancy says that each day he had a little less energy.

"I was harping on him," she said. "But he was struggling and I didn't know it."

By Thursday, June 22, five days after the three-year anniversary visit, Gordon's breathing was becoming more and more difficult. In fact, he surrendered to using oxygen constantly. That night, he called Nancy and finally conceded that it might not be a bad idea to seek admission for pulmonary rehabilitation.

Nancy picked him up the next morning at 7 a.m. for the ninety-minute drive from Pentwater to Spectrum Health in Grand Rapids. She says that she had to dress him and comb his hair. Just north of Muskegon, she called JaNae and described Gordon's condition. JaNae suggested they head straight to ER.

"Something alarmed me in her voice," Nancy recalled. "By that point, Gordon was literally crashing in the car. He was clammy and all slumped over. I was going 90 miles per hour and weaving in and out of cars."

She made the normal ninety-minute trip in a little over an hour. When they arrived, Gordon was unconscious and his clothes had to be cut from his body. Gordon underwent a battery of tests and was admitted to the ICU. His arterial blood gasses were triple the normal limit.

Nancy stayed with Gordon and nervously awaited the conversation with Gordon's pulmonology team. A flurry of questions swirled in her mind. Would he have to be admitted for eighteen days again? Would the blood gasses affect his behavior and personality as they had back in April? Would he face long-term inpatient rehabilitation this time? What would be his quality of life upon discharge? Would they have to spend the entire summer in and out of hospitals?

When Dr. Hadley arrived, he took her down to a family consulting room off the main waiting area, and the questions poured out of her.

Dr. Hadley looked at her strangely, she recalls, and said, "Nancy, this is end of life. Gordon is not coming out of this."

"He was kind, but matter-of-fact," she said. "I literally doubled over and hit the floor. It was total devastation.

"I was beside myself," Nancy said. "Furious and upset—and I had so many questions. Did Gordon know this the whole time? Couldn't someone have told me?"

About 1,400 lung transplants are performed in the United States every year, and about 90 percent of those patients will live at least one year after the procedure. However, only about 55 percent of patients survive five years after transplant, with many suffering from chronic rejection, which causes the airways of the lungs to deteriorate. Gordon had faced chronic rejection issues in addition to his Alpha-1 and chronic obstructive pulmonary disease.

Nancy was aware of the statistics, but said she still always believed Gordon was destined to be a survivor. Now, she had to prepare herself for a hospital stay and for a life that was about to become very different than what she had anticipated.

Nancy spent Friday night at the hospital without getting much sleep. On Saturday, she faced a number of difficult conversations, the first, in person with Gordon and his physicians, and many others by phone advising close friends and family that the end was near. How near, she could not be certain. She had seen Gordon decline and improve on several occasions.

"I thought we might have days or weeks," she recalled. "I couldn't be sure how much time we had left."

She called Gordon's sister, Margo, who visited on Saturday and as many of Gordon's legion of friends as she could—those from Holland and Pentwater, Key West, and those dispersed throughout the world.

Finally she sat down with the hospitalist and staff from palliative care, whose job was to make Gordon as comfortable as possible in his last days and hours.

She had spoken with Gordon throughout Saturday, but his arterial blood gasses were once again high and he passed in and out of consciousness and delirium. Nancy asked a physician from palliative care to accompany her as she sat down and explained things to Gordon.

"I asked the doctor to sit with me and help explain it," she said. "He was so good—not flowery. He was very kind, but matter-of-fact. He told Gordon that he was not coming out of it this time and explained his options."

That day and night, friends, family, and well-wishers came and went. Nancy sat in on many of the conversations. Gordon was on full oxygen with a breathing tube, though he would nod in response to questions.

"The last night I told him God loved him and so did I," said Gordon's sister Margo. "He acknowledged everybody who came to visit him. Their presence meant a lot to him."

"I remember asking him, 'Are you scared?'" Nancy said. "He nodded yes. He had a great fear of not being able to breathe."

Good friends Dave and Kathy Spitler from Pentwater were the last to arrive that night, at about 10:30 p.m. As Nancy and the Spitlers sat and talked to Gordon, Nancy remembers the heart monitor spiking and wondering if each beat might be his last.

"By the time we arrived, he couldn't talk, his blood pressure was going off the charts, and the doctors were trying to determine what to give him," Dave Spitler recalled.

"He was pulling his mask off, was very agitated, and wanted to say something, but he couldn't get enough oxygen into his lungs to get anything out," he added. "I talked to him after they settled him down and told him, 'Don't struggle.'"

The Spitlers said goodbye at about 12:45 a.m. Toward the end of their visit, it had become apparent that Gordon was ready to let go. Nancy asked him if he was ready and he finally nodded yes.

At about 1:15 a.m., Nancy said her last goodbyes and Gordon was given a morphine drip, as had been agreed. After he lost consciousness, his oxygen was removed. Gordon lapsed into a coma for about 20 minutes and was declared dead at 1:52 a.m. on Sunday,

June 25, the day that Fred would begin his participation in the World Transplant Games in Malaga, Spain.

On Sunday, June 25, 2017, exactly three years and one week after receiving his heart transplant, Fred stood alone, with intensely mixed feelings, as the late afternoon shadows gathered outside the Plaza de Toros de La Malagueta, in Malaga, Spain, preparing for the opening ceremonies of the World Transplant Games.

Combined with the feelings of triumph, gratitude, and love for his extended family, many of whom had made the trip to see him compete, were other feelings: thoughts of an anonymous donor who had made this moment possible and to whom his first medal would be dedicated.

And even more poignant, just a few hours earlier, he had received a text from Nancy with the news of Gordon's death. Although not entirely unexpected, the news hit him hard.

"I fully expected to see Gordon after I got back to celebrate with him. Here I am in Spain, just getting ready to celebrate with a bunch of other folks and my kindred spirit passed away.

"That's one of the bittersweet ironies of a gathering like the World Transplant Games," Fred said afterward. "We are all living on borrowed time, but for a transplant recipient, that realization is even more concentrated. Look around. A certain percentage of this year's competitors will not be around to compete next time.

"Gordon had so many more things he wanted to do, so many more projects to undertake, so many more places he wanted to explore," Fred recalled. "Even near the end, Gord was planning out his and Nancy's adventures for the upcoming year, including a repeat of his sailing trip to the South Pole.

"You could see Gordon's pride and determination just a week prior to his passing," he added, referring to the visit we had all made the previous week to celebrate the three-year anniversary of their transplants. "I'm glad we got to see him on a bittersweet three-year anniversary.

"We weren't brothers, but we were comingled spirits," Fred said. "He had his personality quirks as I do, but we were an interesting couple, an odd couple for sure."

BACK AT THE OPENING CEREMONIES

As thoughts of Gordon and of his anonymous donor whirled through his mind, Fred tried to focus on the road he had taken to get here.

"I went to the Games as a transplant recipient to celebrate life, but in addition, as an athlete to compete and see how I would stack up to others who were also there to compete," Fred recalled later.

The World Transplant Games Federation, established in 1978, is a worldwide organization with representation from more than sixty countries that celebrates successful transplantation and the gift of life through unique and inspiring events—namely the Summer and Winter World Transplant Games.

Fred's training for Malaga had begun in earnest on August 15, 2014, 57 days after transplant. His first practice was 1,100 yards and took 40 minutes to finish. Over the course of the next 34 months, he swam 1,426,350 yards or 810 miles. Taking into account travel to and from the Holland Community Aquatic Center as well as locker room time, his training commitment totaled about 15 hours per week.

There were no complaints or regrets running through Fred's mind, just the hope that this training would pay off at the Games.

"Athletes second guess themselves all the time," Fred said. "'Did I do enough? Did I do too much?' After starting up in August, I had delusions of grandeur. Some practices were so demanding it was all I could do to just find the energy to get dressed."

Fred was still dealing with a number of physical ailments, including the continuation of "stiff heart," which put him at a competitive disadvantage to swimmers recovering from, say, liver or kidney transplants. There was also the matter of the damage to his phrenic nerve, which had yet to completely heal, and the thoracic outlet syndrome in his left arm that still plagued him. Suffice it to say that, in addition to his grief, Fred was anxious. He didn't know what to expect, competing at this level.

THE OPENING CEREMONIES began late and the teams made their entry into the Plaza de Toros, one-by-one, in alphabetical order by country.

Fred waited outside the stadium, lined up with his United States teammates behind most of the other 52 countries. These included large delegations from Great Britain, Spain, Germany, and the US, with scores of participants and supporters, and smaller teams, some with only one, or a handful of participants, such as those from India, Lebanon, and Morocco.

These 2500 athletes, ranging in age from youth to age 90, all of whom had either donated kidneys or bone marrow or received lifesaving transplants of heart, lungs, liver, pancreas, kidneys, and/or bone marrow, would spend the next week engaged in friendly competition.

Each team received a rousing ovation as its athletes made the full circuit of the stadium, celebrating the moment and awaiting the start of the next day's preliminary events in cycling, track and field, volleyball, kayaking, basketball, and the triathlon. Other events included badminton, bowling, darts, golf, squash, table tennis, Petanque, and of course, swimming, which would get underway on Wednesday.

Fred finally made his way into the Plaza in the early evening, after sweating in the 90-degree heat for more than two hours. He was the very last member of the US team to enter, taking his time, hat off and waving to his loved ones, taking photos of the crowd and his teammates, savoring the moment. He was fully aware of what his participation meant to him and to his loved ones. He was also thinking of an anonymous donor, and of his kindred spirit, Gordon Veldman.

Malaga would be very different from Cleveland in one way: he and Jean had chosen not to fly solo this time. In fact, they had made good on Fred's promise of a family vacation by paying the way for a veritable entourage. In addition to Jean, his four daughters, Kelly Nicholas, Heather Dykstra, Lindsey Rocafort, and Jami Nelis had made the trip along with their husbands, Ryan Nicholas, Colt Dykstra, Sergio Rocafort, and Jami's fiancé, Derrick Taylor. Fred's sister, Charlotte Nelis, was also in attendance as were three old family friends, Jill Caesar and John and Karen Steuber as well as Sergio's brother and sister-in-law, José Luis and Mimi Rocafort. The Dykstras' five-month-old daughter, Willamena, rounded out the fan club.

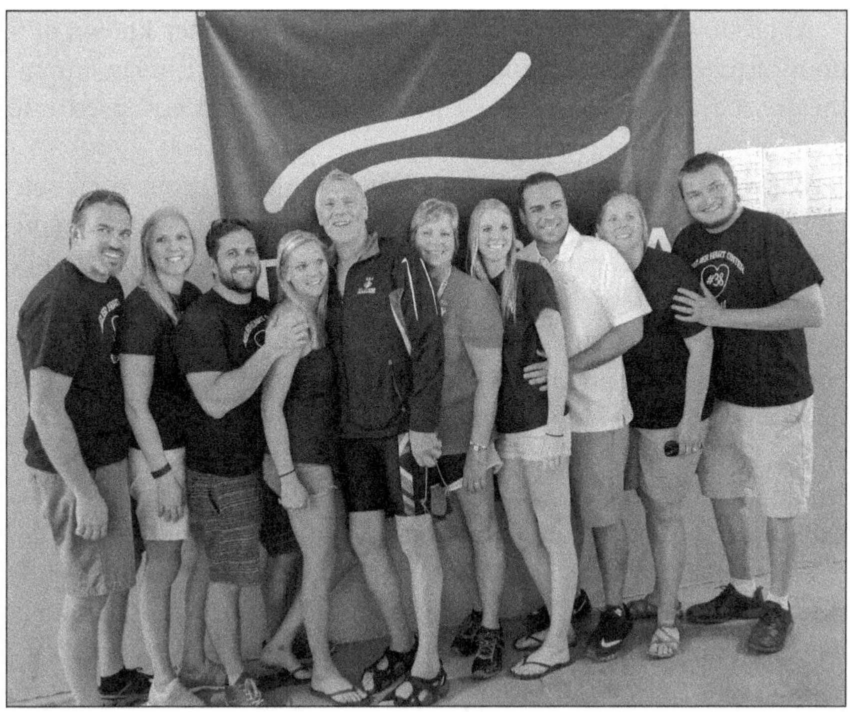

Nelis family pic Malaga Spain

After every nation's team had entered the stadium, the evening's largest round of applause was reserved for the parade of donors and donor families. It was an emotional outpouring of thanks from the individuals who had been given the gift of life to those who had helped to make that gift possible.

AN UNEXPECTED SETBACK

At dinner that night, sick with a cold, jet-lagged, and dehydrated, Fred was low-key. He was thinking about the day's events and the 48 hours he had to get ready to compete in the 50-meter backstroke, the 50-meter butterfly, and the 50-, 100-, and 200-meter freestyle events.

As he stood to leave El Pimpi, one of Malaga's better-known out-door restaurants, located in a plaza fronting the old Roman amphi-theatre, he staggered, knocked over the table, and collapsed into Jean's arms.

With the help of several bystanders, he was lifted, unconscious, onto an empty table. The restaurant's owner fanned his face with an *abanico*, the traditional Spanish fan borrowed from a female patron, while a waiter held his legs above his head and an ambulance was called.

After his vital signs checked out, Fred was advised by Spanish paramedics to rest and to remember to hydrate throughout the long dry days under the hot sun on Spain's Costa del Sol.

The Games would begin Monday, the following morning, but he would have until Wednesday to recuperate and to get his blood pressure under control before the swimming events got underway.

Although Jean had learned not to underestimate her husband's determination, she was very concerned as she watched Fred slump, exhausted, into the taxi that would take them back to their hotel. She wondered if, perhaps, they had made the long trip for nothing.

"It was an emotional roller coaster," Jean recalled. "It's a fragile balance for a transplant patient and you can tip the cart easily. You kind of forget that sometimes."

WEDNESDAY: SWIMMERS, TAKE YOUR MARKS

Even in the best environments, a swim competition can be hot, crowded, and noisy.

In the enclosed space of the Centro Acuatico de Malaga on Wednesday morning, boisterous chanting made for a clamorous crowd. Fans of the Argentine and Brazilian swimmers were espe-cially exuberant, lending to an atmosphere more akin to soccer's World Cup.

Fred's family, no strangers to natatoriums, took it all in with delight.

"He's always been a swimmer," said Jean. "When he had the LVAD and he couldn't get wet, he felt so bad. He always wanted to get back in the pool. And a transplant was the way to do that."

"That was the goal from the start—to always be able to come back and swim," their youngest daughter, Jami, said. "Both parents have always been there for us and have always been our biggest cheerleaders, so it's great to be able to do that now for him."

For his part, Fred felt much better.

He knew he'd be diving into a flurry of competitors, each bearing the scars of transplant. Many had the names of donors and surgery dates written proudly in marker across their backs and torsos.

Mingled with that competitive vibe was an unmistakable sense of gratitude and respect.

"Everybody here has been through hell in their lives," Jean said. "And they are happy to be healthy. A new kind of healthy. And happy to be here."

"The amount of love in this group is humbling," said Lindsey. "Everyone has their common person to support, but it is also the camaraderie of the situation that heightens everything."

Jean, meanwhile, worried secretly about her husband's health, despite the brave front she maintained for her family.

"I keep telling him, 'You need to drink, you need to eat, you need to adjust your medications,'" she said.

Fred's first day of competition came with surprises—some pleasant, some unpleasant.

In the 200-meter freestyle, he took fourth place, finishing behind gold medalist Chikara Wakamatsu, of Japan.

Fred would come to recognize that name well over the next two days.

In the 50-meter backstroke, not typically one of his better races, Fred surprised himself and his family with a strong second-place finish, gliding in just behind Great Britain's Simon Randerson.

Fred dedicated that medal to his anonymous heart donor.

"There isn't a lot more you can say to the donor family," Fred said. "Three years of effort have gone into this. My note is just going to say,

'Thank you.' There are just no words to express your gratitude to a family that parted with their loved one."

His family's sentiments were evident.

"I'm pretty proud," said Kelly. "It was a little emotional, but fun to see. Dad's been to about a thousand of my swim meets—and it's nice to be able to go to one of his."

"They definitely were at every swim meet that I ever had," said Jami. "He really tries to take advantage of this new opportunity after this heart transplant, it made him more determined he was going to swim at the Games, celebrate this new life. He was swimming for both Gordon and himself at that point, as motivation to be able to do his best."

SPIRIT OF COMPETITION

As Wednesday progressed, Fred also won silver in the 50-meter butterfly. Once again, he finished just behind Wakamatsu.

The day's final race, the 100-meter freestyle, was historically one of Fred's stronger competitions, and he got off to a good start, keeping pace much of the first lap.

After the turn, however, two swimmers began to pull away. A late kick put Fred next to the swimmer in the lane to his left, Lu Jin Xiang, of China. Both men appeared to slap the wall simultaneously, but the official time showed Xiang edging Fred for the silver medal and Fred had to settle for the bronze.

On Thursday, Fred would get one more chance at Wakamatsu, in a showdown in the 50-meter freestyle.

Fred's final event demanded a no-holds-barred race from one end of the pool to the other. No holding back. No saving energy for a final kick. No hopeful spurt to overcome the leader.

As the bell sounded, both swimmers got off to a strong start. Fred's strong, fluid strokes propelled him along lane 5. Wakamatsu kept pace in lane 4.

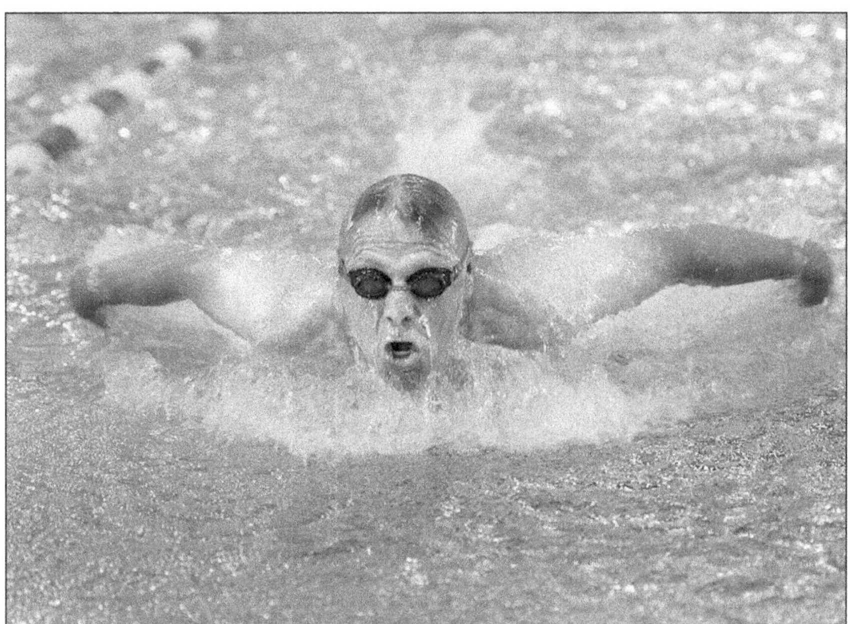

Fred butterfly stroke

At the halfway point, it appeared the two were neck and neck. Both swam several body lengths ahead of the nearest competitor. As Fred and Wakamatsu cruised toward the finish, it looked, from Jean's angle, like a dead heat.

Both swimmers appeared to touch the wall simultaneously. As the two men leaned over the ropes to shake hands, the official time showed Wakamatsu the winner by three-tenths of a second. The gold would elude Fred this year.

After his final race, he found the awaiting arms of his family.

"I'm ecstatic," Jean said. "I'm much more relaxed. He's done great. I didn't realize I was nervous, but now that it is over, I'm relieved."

Fred felt relieved, but perhaps a little motivated too.

The 2019 World Transplant Games were slated for Newcastle, England.

"We'll have to see," Fred said, mulling the idea. "I tried very hard, but there are a lot of talented swimmers here."

22

The Sailor:
Fair Winds and a Following Sea

"It's strange how a person who embraced life in giant gulps, who was the epitome of a breath of fresh air, was taken because his lungs, that in essence are kind of a carburetor to take in and mix oxygen into the blood that fuels the engine that makes our bodies live, failed him."

—STEVE BEGNOCHE

PENTWATER LAKE is a sparkling blue jewel that gives the town that shares its name a reason to exist. Fed by north and south branches of the Pentwater River, into which flow a number of smaller tributaries such as Watson, Cedar, and Dumaw Creeks, the lake's deepest point is only 50 feet. But, like many bodies of water in the region, the lake's west end connects via channel to the depths of Lake Michigan.

The venerable Pentwater Yacht Club sits along the lake's northwest shore in the heart of town, not far from the channel leading out to the boundless waters of the greater world. Located just down the hill from his abode, which overlooks the lake, Gordon spent many days and nights at the club over the years, keeping up with old friends, making new ones, and as always, regaling the assembled crew with his treasure trove of experience and stories. On the afternoon of September 24, 2017, dozens of his friends, admirers, and loved ones gathered at the club for a celebration of life to pay their final respects and to recall their memories of time well-spent in Gordon's company.

It was a warm and sunny Sunday in Pentwater. A craft fair and market took place throughout downtown that day, and between the fair and Gordon's celebration, it was hard to find parking within six blocks of the yacht club. But that didn't stop those coming to pay their respects. In fact, the celebration had been set in motion for several months following his death on June 25, with best wishes and bon voyage already setting sail down the Missouri River in the form of a "Spirit Boat."

Adopted from a Japanese Buddhist ritual to mourn the recent dead, a small, handmade boat, decorated with the family crest, a portrait, and perhaps a token to symbolize the deceased, is launched into a river and out to sea. The boats are said to carry the souls of the dead and are mainly built by people who have lost a family member in the past year.

Gordon's friends, Peg and Kent Gage, who had planned a mid-September camping trip that would take them to the banks of the Mississippi and Missouri Rivers, came up with the idea to pay tribute to their friend. Throughout the summer, the Gages and Nancy collected dozens of short descriptions of Gordon from friends and well-wishers to inscribe onto the boat. These included: "courageous, curiosity, engaging, free-spirit, instructive, invigorating, lasagna, original, wise, woodworker, and *Just Dandy*."

In a close approximation of Gordon and Carol's 1980 sailing adventure, the Gages launched the boat from the banks of Council Bluffs, Iowa, out onto the Missouri River with the hope that it would eventually flow into the mighty Mississippi and find its way to open sea.

"We had talked about the Mississippi but went with the Missouri because it was a major part of our Lewis and Clark Trail expedition, and we thought it honored Gordon's spirit of adventure and exploration," Kent Gage explained.

ON THE DAY of the Celebration of Life, the yacht club was decked out with photos and mementos of Gordon as family and friends from far and wide mingled, sharing memories and stories.

Gordon's brother, Tom, sister Margo, and other relatives mingled with friends from his Holland days, his Pentwater days, and from his travels. Many, such as Greg and Barb Siewert, now living in Seattle, traveled great distances to be there.

"Gordon taught me how to love life," Greg Siewert said. "He was a true friend and I wouldn't have missed it for the world."

The Gordon stories flowed and sometimes gushed forth, as easily and unstoppable as fair winds and a following sea, both during informal conversations and the formal part of the program where many stepped forth to eulogize him. Many of the tales have already been told throughout the pages of this book, and some elicited tears, though most ended in laughter.

After everyone had settled in with food and drink in hand, Nancy welcomed the assembled guests with loving memories of Gordon.

"Friends and family meant the world to him," she said.

She recalled their times together snowshoeing, kayaking, traveling, and cozying up with maple syrup and a bottle of rum on a cold spring morning in the Vartians' sugar shack.

"When we say we were soulmates, we were soulmates," she said. "His passing has affected me tremendously. He opened me up to a whole different world."

Gordon's friend, Joe Clark, who had taken the photograph of the Transplant Brothers that went viral, served as master of ceremonies of the remembrance period, during which those gathered were invited to pay tribute to Gordon.

"Gordon lived a life most of us don't get to experience, that the rest of us can only aspire to," he said in his remarks, before sharing Gordon's theory of sailing in a storm (which is worth repeating):

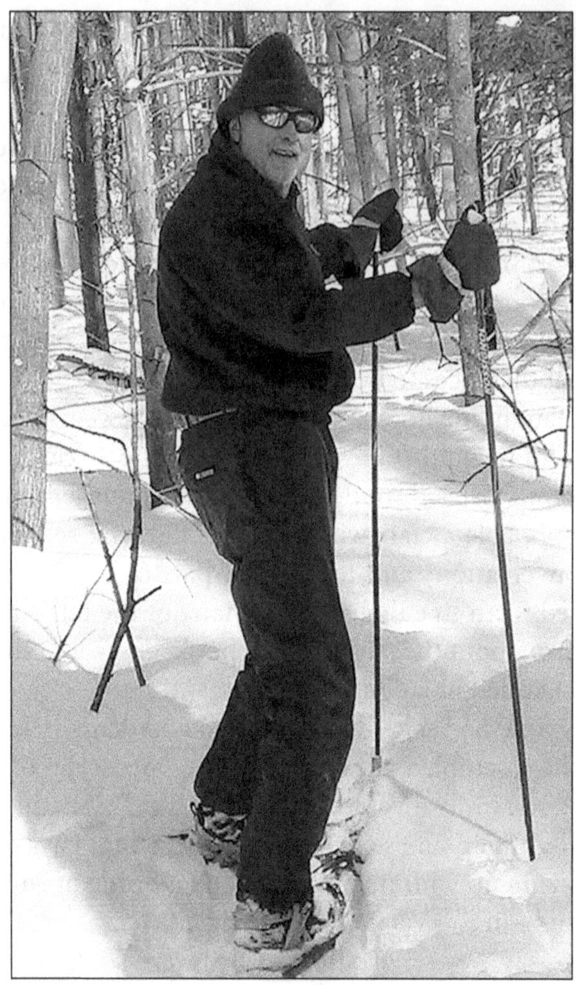

Gordon snowshoeing

"Either you get hit by lightning or you don't. If you get hit by lightning, either you live or you don't. And in any case, you have a great story to tell."

Greg Siewert recalled a visit from Gordon when they took their bikes down to Mexico's Baja Peninsula, racing downhill from Tijuana to Ensenada just as fast as they could go, oblivious to the potholed Mexican roads.

He also added another anecdote about three large men (Gordon, John Vande Bunte, and Steve Wolff again) shooting off fireworks from a floating raft on Bills Lake: "It was a great show, but I do recall some singed clothes."

Chrissie Hall shared a number of memories of sailing the North Channel with Gordon, including the time they used a bag of Fritos as fuel for a fire, as well as recollections of the great belly-dancing birthday trick perpetrated on an unsuspecting friend, detailed earlier.

Gordon's brother, Tom, recalled Gordon's penchant for smoke bombs and blowing things up as a child and the Pontiac Trans Am with racing slicks he drove as a teenager.

Beverly Fogarty stepped to the microphone about midway through the ceremony.

"I think most of you know who I am," said the woman who had been with Gordon the longest.

She shared the funny story of their wild bicycle ride through the rain on Cape Breton Island, as well as a gentler recollection of that trip.

"We were camped out in a farmer's field and a little old lady invited us in for bacon, eggs, and orange juice," she said. "We were grateful, because we were out of food and there was nothing but rocks, trees, and water. It was gorgeous."

It is telling that on the day of Gordon's Celebration of Life, Nancy mingled freely with Beverly, who had become a good friend, as well as several other ex-lovers and girlfriends—all of whom joined in raising a good-spirited toast.

"Bev and I agree that he had great taste in women," Nancy said.

Heide Kenjorski recalled the first time she met Gordon and being impressed by his ability to recite the entirety of Robert Service's 15-stanza ballad, "The Cremation of Sam McGee," from memory.

This recollection elicited groans and boos from some who had apparently heard the recitation more than a few times.

Although Gordon had no children, he did have a fondness for young people and a special way with them. Many discussed his enthusiasm for sharing science experiments with classrooms of school children. One-on-one he was just as charming.

A young woman, whose mother had lived with Gordon in the 1980s, recalled the trapeze in the living room, but also shared memories of handmade wooden toys, a play room with a doll house, a baby possum, and ice skating behind Gordon's ice boat.

"He was very influential in my life," she said. "I used to pray that my mother would marry him."

A niece, Missy Hewitt, posted on Gordon's obituary page:

"What great memories of my Uncle Gord that I will cherish from my childhood all the way up to present. I will forever think of Pentwater as 'Gord's place'! I love you Uncle Gord and will miss you. XO."

Toward the end of the public remembrance, Fred stood up to speak.

"We had one of the most unique relationships in the room," he started, recalling his final visit with Gordon on June 17. "He didn't want to say goodbye, but I had an inkling that might be the case."

He recalled finding out about Gordon's death from Nancy on the day of the opening ceremonies in Malaga and reflecting on the three extra years of life that Gordon's transplant afforded him.

"It was a second act for Gordon," he said. "He sailed, he raked the leaves, he rode his bike, he found the love of his life in Nancy.

"It's not how far you go in life," he added. "It's how fast you go far. And there are few people who could cram as much living and celebrating life into three years as Gordon was able to do."

A sobbing Kayla Clark, Joe Clark's wife, took the mic with her husband's arm around her.

"I've probably known him the shortest amount of time of anyone here…I wish I'd known him longer," she said. "He has helped me much, and is the greatest man I have ever met in my life. I hope I get to meet more, but Gordon will probably top them all."

One of the last people to speak, a middle-aged man, said, "I'm so glad to stay here telling his stories. I'm going to leave here channeling Gordon…We are all still connected."

AFTER THE CELEBRATION, a number of friends, led by Joe Clark, were reluctant to let go of the mood of reminiscence and so decamped to Gordon's house just up the hill from the yacht club, where the stories continued long into the night.

Dave and Kim Wildner, Gordon's next-door neighbors throughout the early 1990s, had recently moved back to the area with the hopes of rekindling their friendship.

"He was one of the first who reached out and reconnected when we got back to Michigan," Kim Wildner wrote in a Facebook post. "And we easily fell into the same old comfortable conversations. We looked forward to spending more time together.

"But time is such a precious thing and he had so little," she added. "In true Gordon fashion he filled it to the brim."

Instead, the Wildners would be entrusted with the ownership of *Just Dandy*, which would ferry Gordon's ashes to the first of three final planned resting places: Pentwater Lake, within sight of Gordon's house along the northeast shore. The rest of his ashes were to later be scattered in two other places he held dear: the North Channel of Lake Huron and the Florida Keys.

As his loved ones reluctantly filed out of the yacht club, Nancy readied Gordon's remains for a sunset cruise she would take along with Dave Wildner and friends Terry and Mary Ann Boom.

"We were teary-eyed putting him back where he wanted to be," Nancy later recalled. "Right in front of his home, but in the water."

"*Just Dandy* set sail and said goodbye to her only commander since her maiden voyage," Dave Wildner wrote afterward in a Facebook post. "Now, I have the honor and responsibility of sailing her into the future, and with a final tribute to our dear friend, as we sailed past his longtime nest following the beautiful celebration of his life. Rest in Peace, dear Gordon, you will be missed."

"It's so great Gordon is sailing in waters he so much loved," commented longtime friend, Wendy Ryder.

In the end, Nancy was unable to bring herself to scatter Gordon's remaining ashes so far from home.

"I took the remainder of his ashes and spread them in front of my house on the shores of Lake Michigan on his birthday, November 28," she said. "I wanted him near me and decided not to do the Key West or North Channel spots."

IN ADDITION TO his immediate family, Gordon's obituary included mention of his soulmate, Nancy, his cat, Ralphie (adopted by a friend), and his transplant brother, Fred Nelis. He would also be memorialized in print by others.

Longtime friend Steve Begnoche wrote a column for the *Ludington Daily News* called "Take time for what's really important," in which he upbraided himself for postponing a pot roast dinner with Gordon and Nancy until it was too late:

"Last summer he and Nancy got to use the cottage (where Begnoche had installed ash boards that Gordon had planed and given to him)…He said he was pleased with how the ash was used, much of it to trim out the porch I was sitting in when I read of Gordon's passing…Gordon will always be a part of our life in ways more important than porch trim and pot roast. Yet there's something appropriate about the wood being in the room that, like Gordon, enjoys breezes from the lake during summer and braves the chill of winter."

Writing in *Oceana's Herald Journal*, Mary Beth Crain also paid homage to Gordon:

"Gordon charmed me from the beginning. With his longish gray hair and beard, rosy cheeks and beaming smile, he looked a little like Santa's tall, skinny brother. He was a wonderful interview, his humor and candor enriched by an all-encompassing knowledge of everything from science, politics and the arts to canning peppers, making Limoncello and baking that classic Dutch pastry, *banket*. Above all, he was an inspiration—a man so delighted with his second chance at life that he was determined to pack as much as he could into every drop of every day."

23

"...Soar Like an Eagle"

A S 2018 HEADS TO A CLOSE, the Richard DeVos Heart & Lung Transplant Program continues its hectic pace toward further milestones under the medical leadership of Drs. Boeve, Dickinson, and Girgis. Rahn Bentley's first-ever transplant in 2010 and even Fred's heart transplant (the Transplant Program's 38th) now seem a long way in the rearview mirror as the program continues to provide a last chance for those in need of a lifesaving option.

Transplant "lifers" Becky Shore and Krista Veine also continue their work as managers in the program, but there have been changes. Dr. Asghar Khaghani has returned to England to work as a semi-retired, consulting transplant surgeon. On his very last day at Spectrum Health, on May 26, 2017, I had the honor of presenting Dr. Khaghani with the T-shirt Fred had made to celebrate his upcoming participation in the World Transplant Games in Malaga.

As we sat in a conference room on the 8th floor of the Spectrum Heart Meijer Heart Center, we spoke to Fred via speaker phone and I watched Dr. Khaghani fold the T-shirt very carefully and tenderly with his skilled surgeon's hands, one small fold after another.

"I'm very proud to have been a part of your stay here in Michigan," Fred's voice crackled over the speaker, his gratitude to the man who had performed his lifesaving surgery evident even in the absence of his smiling countenance.

"Thank you very much," Khaghani responded. "I will look at this from time to time and feel very proud."

There have been other changes. After twenty-one years of living with a transplanted heart, Richard DeVos, the entrepreneur and philanthropist who gave the Spectrum Health transplant program its name and helped to jumpstart an economic renaissance in his hometown, passed away September 6, 2018, at age 92. His impact on the West Michigan community was huge.

"Rich DeVos leaves a lasting legacy that will continue to benefit countless people through improved health care quality and access," said Dr. Richard McNamara, DeVos's longtime cardiologist and founding co-director of Spectrum Health's Frederik Meijer Heart & Vascular Institute.

"Rich's generosity is helping to enable advanced treatments and a better quality of life for patients in West Michigan who used to have no option close to home and family," he added.

Before Rich DeVos passed away, Fred was able to fulfill a long-held wish to send him a gift of thanks for his role in creating the transplant program that gave him and Gordon and many others a second chance. Fred helped write and design a small commemorative book about his experience, and together with a medal won at the World Transplant Games in Malaga 2017, and a hand-written letter, was able to convey his gratitude to a man he considers to be a titan of industry and philanthropy.

"Mr. DeVos gave back to both the hometown that nurtured him and to the transplant community with which he shared the attitude of gratitude," Fred said. "We can't all contribute vast sums of money or use our business acumen to move mountains, but each survivor must be willing to contribute whatever we are able for the common good and to honor the memory of our donors."

WHAT THE FUTURE HOLDS

Despite the growth of transplant programs and technological advances in transplant surgery and organ recovery, a constant shortage of suitable organs continues throughout the nation and the world. As of publication, there remain nearly 114,000 people in the US on waiting lists for organ transplants. More than 7,000 people on those lists each year likely will not live to receive one.

Scientists continue to make breakthroughs in many areas, including xenotransplantation, chimeras, regenerative medicine, 3D-printed organs, bio-artificial approaches, and mechanical devices such as VADs. Despite the host of medical and technological breakthroughs, other experts feel that the organ shortage crisis will not be solved in the laboratory or operating room, but in the halls of the legislature and policymaking organizations.

Our fifty states currently operate an "opt-in" approach to organ donation, which requires potential donors to provide consent by signing up—online, in person, or when renewing a driver's license. Conversely, "opt-out" organ donation operates on the principle of "presumed consent," implying that everyone is a potential donor unless they sign up to remove themselves from the list. Different versions of opt-out programs already exist in two dozen European countries including Spain, Belgium, and France. A 2012 Stanford and Cornell study found that organ donation rates are "typically exceeding 90 percent in opt-out countries and failing to reach even 15 percent in opt-in countries."

A number of states including Connecticut, Texas, Colorado, and Pennsylvania, have introduced legislation to convert their organ donation processes to an opt-out system, but none of these bills have advanced into law.

Michigan undertook a simple policy change that has led to a huge increase in the donor registry. Through a coordinated effort between Michigan Gift of Life and the Secretary of State's office, when someone renews their driver's license at a branch of the Secretary of State, a computer prompt will not allow the employee to complete a registration until the applicant has been asked if he or she would like to sign up for the organ donation registry. Previously, it was left up to the employee to ask the question. This small change has tripled the registry to include 66 percent of Michigan adults in just a few years.

This easy fix is in keeping with the essential message of this story: For the time being, the greatest difference any individual can make remains becoming an organ donor. It is easy, painless, and free, takes only a matter of minutes, and can make all the difference in the world.

When families and loved ones are taken into the equation, the impact is exponential.

As scientists, clinicians, citizen advocates, and policymakers forge ahead to find solutions to the organ shortage crisis, donors, recipients, and family members also continue to forge ahead. Some are blessed by a loved one with a new chance at life, and others continue on in their absence, striving to bring meaning to their sacrifice.

CATCHING UP WITH DONORS, FAMILY MEMBERS, AND OTHERS

Nancy's days have changed without the love of her life at her side, but she is reminded on a constant basis of the difference that knowing Gordon has made to her life.

"I led a very ordered life and did not take risks at all," she said. "I would never have done half of the things or even thought of half the things I have done without Gordon in my life."

"I am better," she said. "But I have my moments."

A day of remembrance at the Unitarian Universalist Church in Ludington was difficult. She tries to stay busy: traveling with her friends, dog-walking, and volunteering for the local animal shelter, using her accounting background to prepare tax returns for the elderly as tax season rolls around, and working on her creative writing, which she has had some success publishing.

In the months following Gordon's death, one of her sisters came to stay with her for a few months, which helped take her mind off missing him.

One of the biggest reminders of Gordon on a daily basis is trying to figure out how to ration the last of the canned food he left behind. Every time she opens a jar and catches a whiff of its contents, it is another reminder of Gordon.

"I'm hanging on to his homemade salsa like gold," she said. "I only have two jars left."

She has about fifty quarts of his home-canned grape juice, but she knows that even these will not last indefinitely.

Nancy tries her best to stay in touch with Gordon's myriad of friends and says many have gone out of their way to include her in activities in the year following his death. She was delighted to report in late 2018 that Kayla and Joe Clark are expecting their first child. If the baby is a boy, the Clarks have decided to name him Gordon.

CATCHING UP WITH FRED

"Catching up" is probably not the best choice of words to describe Fred's progress throughout 2018 and into Salt Lake City, because few were able to keep pace with him. At the 2018 TGA event, he swam faster than his previous competitions by one to two seconds in every event he competed in, and he nearly had to pay an extra baggage fee to fly home all of the hardware he won.

His results included gold medals in the 50-yard freestyle, 100-yard freestyle, 50-yard fly, 50-yard backstroke, 200-yard medley relay and 200-yard freestyle relay; He won silver in the 200-yard individual medley and the 500-yard freestyle.

As successful as he continued to be in sprint events, Fred felt it was his finishes in the two distance events that really marked the next step in his transformation from transplant patient to well-rounded competitive swimmer.

But even more exciting and fulfilling to Fred than the results were some of the physical and psychological changes he experienced that led to his success. The thoracic outlet syndrome that had plagued him throughout the games in Cleveland and Malaga was much more manageable.

"I had plenty of that in Cleveland and in Spain," he said. "The blood supply doesn't get to the arm muscle. But somehow I reduced its effects, perhaps by stretching and changing my stroke a little bit."

Another thing that he left in his wake was the pre-competition doubt that plagued him in his first meets, post-transplant.

"Contrasting the Cleveland Transplant Games in 2016 with the Salt Lake Games was a night and day difference," he said. "I wanted to race instead of dreading to race. That's the athlete coming back. The juices that flowed when I was a good swimmer returned."

"It is a huge learning curve," he added. "There are no textbooks or Google Maps. It just takes a lot of time."

Fred made it to the 2019 World Transplant Games in Newcastle, England. He won gold in the 50-meter backstroke, 50 freestyle, 100 backstroke, and 200 free mixed relay. He also won silver in the 100 freestyle.

Following the games, Jean and Fred along with John and Karen Steuber, as well as Fred's college roommate John MacArthur and his wife Gail, celebrated Gordwardian style: they "set sail" and spent nine days traveling by boat up the Rhine River before returning to reality and work.

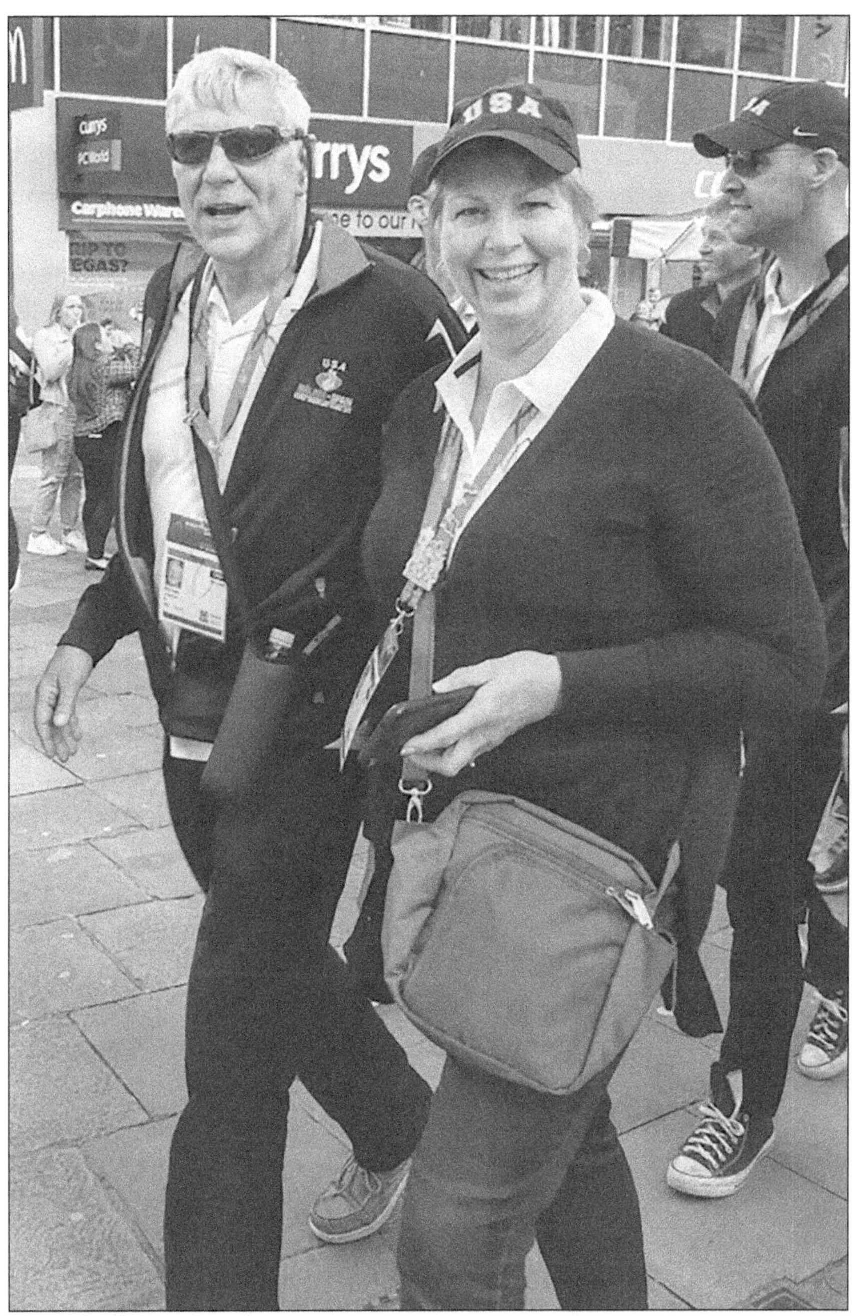

Fred and Jean in the Newcastle parade

"REACH: STOP TRYING TO LIVE, START LIVING TO TRY."

It has been stated and repeated that Fred is a man of contradictions—one who carries the weight of moral responsibility and gratitude on his shoulders, one who sets out to honor in every way possible an individual he has never met, one who lives every day with the need to prove that he is worthy of a great gift, that his donor did not die in vain.

Those who know him best have referred to him throughout this story as "relentless, a workhorse, mentally disciplined, determined, competitive, the leader of the pack," and one who "plays the cards you are dealt."

Yet that overwhelming sense of obligation does not make him glum, overly serious, or self-absorbed. Quite the opposite.

He is also referred to by those same friends and loved ones as: "generous," "a connector," someone who "doesn't give up on you," "a bigger-than-life character," "crazy, with a very unusual sense of humor," who, even when sick "cared about giving the nurses and doctors a good day," who has "brought more joy to the people at Spectrum Health than anyone," and who, even when ill "looks for the positive and for ways to enjoy himself with others."

The hard work, the intensity, the striving for improvement, the long hours of practice, the weight of responsibility and duty all have their part. However, in the end they must all give way and share equal time with the T-shirts, slogans, jokes, smiles, laughter, good times, acceptance, gratitude, generosity, grace under pressure, and strong feeling for others.

It is quite a striking dichotomy. One rarely comes across an individual so driven and intense on the one hand and good-humored, generous, and accepting on the other. Part of it may be explained by his faith and the deeply personal mystical experience that took place on the top floor of Holland Hospital (described in Chapter 19). Part of it is also certainly explained by his upbringing, where he was taught, as his sister Charlotte relates, "You are given your plate and deal with it and do the best you can...It's not about 'poor me' or 'oh woe is me.'"

However, that acceptance did not leave him a passive and compliant invalid. Instead, mixed with faith, courage, and determination, it gave him the strength to defy prevailing wisdom, to challenge his doctors' orders, to seek a second opinion, to know his own body, mind, and soul better than anyone else, and to challenge himself to push himself to the limits, not just to survive, but to thrive.

Fred's "Four F's" of Food, Fun, Friends, and Family (and the fifth one, Faith) are something more than just his swimming philosophy, to some extent illustrating his philosophy of life, as well. He also coined a phrase that echoes the Michael Phelps epigraph at the heading of this chapter, one that serves him as a guiding metaphor for this book and as a philosophy for swimming and living: "Reach: Stop trying to live, start living to try."

Fred will continue to reach, and he will continue to try, as long as he lives and as long as there remain blue skies and open water.

You will find him at all of his accustomed places: in Holland with Jean and their family, at work at Yost Vises, swimming laps at the Holland Community Aquatic Center, at play on his quads up at Black Mountain Lodge. But you may also find him where you least expect to. Don't be surprised if he and Jean finally set out on an additional junket of world travel they've been postponing all these years to work and raise a family.

When it finally comes down to explaining Fred's complex character, those who know him, and those who have read about him, can go round and round about nature v. nurture and the role of faith and upbringing. Several friends, however, have cut straight to the heart of the matter by referencing the 1974 hit song by the group America that describes the Wizard of Oz's Tin Man and his quest for a heart:

"But Oz never did give nothing to the Tin Man, that he didn't already have..."

The Tin Man, or perhaps more appropriately, the Iron Man, shall have the last word:

Salt Lake City was intended to be a stepping stone to challenge, reward, and dream of days past. As a young man my dreams focused on breaking 50 seconds in the 100 yard freestyle. Now my donor and I are setting a goal of breaking 60 seconds for the same distance. Also part of the swimming bucket list is to win an event at the Michigan Masters state meet.

Is there a message here? Yes, and a challenge for those who have received a second chance, a do-over if you will. Recipients are not made of glass, they won't break, but even if they do, be assured that setbacks are part of life. It's just that we may have had a few more than most.

In a sense this book is a challenge to not just those of us who got a second chance, but to all who think that the road is too rocky, the sun too hot, and life too tough.

Reach: Stop trying to live, start living to try.

Afterword

FRED NELIS

IT WAS OUR INTENTION to have had this story available much sooner. Like so many things nothing is ever easy or guaranteed. It's a good feeling that it's finally going to happen.

In the meanwhile:

At the conclusion of the 2019 World Transplant Games (WTG) in England, Jean and I spent additional time in Europe with friends, on a relaxing riverboat cruise. After returning home, Jean was off to Denver to assist daughter Lindsey with the arrival of a baby girl (our second granddaughter and fourth grandchild). Grandpa also visited the latest arrival after things settled down.

You might remember reading, earlier in the book, about our business, Yost Vises. It may surprise the reader, but even after my 42 years of employment and thinking by now everyone should have at least one vise in the garage, we are busier than ever. Apparently, vises and tools continue to be a holiday favorite because our busiest months are usually November, December, and January.

February was also surprisingly busy with work and sales remaining very strong, requiring additional six- and seven-day workweeks.

Then, March of 2020.

Many people, me included, turned our attention to the news from Washington State where an alarming number of people in nursing homes were getting sick and dying. Within a couple of weeks the plague was found in Michigan and the lockdowns began. All nonessential businesses and activities were forced to close for the foreseeable future.

The only silver lining for our company was that as a supplier to the Federal Government we were exempt from state mandates to shutter our business. This was both a relief and cause for concern. As March ended, an explosion occurred with existing e-commerce customers. The stay-at-home mandates were a virtual tsunami for home improvement and hobby activity demand.

While our inventory was adequate for normal business activity, it soon was apparent that demand would outstrip supply. The bulk of Yost's products are made in China, and this would become an issue because the country had already shut down their economy in February. Production didn't resume until April. Even as shipments resumed, it was still another six weeks before products were back in inventory.

The Transplant Games of America were scheduled for July 2020. The thought was to hold the Games in the eastern United States to promote awareness for organ donation. The New Jersey, New York areas have some of the lowest organ donation registration in the country, so the hope was to spur interest by hosting the Games. Of course the Games were postponed and eventually transformed into a virtual event, to be held in the summer of 2021.

As much as I look forward to the Games, I was relieved by the cancellation because the timing was near the height of the pandemic in the metropolitan New York area. Additionally, Michigan had continued restrictions on activities such as pools and gyms. Our local pool was closed in mid-March with no reopening date provided.

With no swimming opportunities available I was hoping to allow my chronically painful right shoulder time to heal. But the pace of work at Yost remained at record levels and the wear and tear of all the heavy lifting dashed any hopes of avoiding further damage to the shoulder. As a distraction to the discomfort of a throbbing shoulder, Memorial Day weekend brought the unwarranted diagnosis of a case of shingles.

Too much work, no swimming, shingles, the lockdowns, and the explosion of Covid-19 just crushed my spirit. I understand my comments make me sound ungrateful, but as an immunosuppressed person there was little or no information being provided about what might or could happen to someone like me if exposed to the disease. I was frustrated, as were many other transplant recipients.

After my transplant in June of 2014, the Clinic wanted recipients to basically follow the health and safety guidelines currently promoted by the CDC. Can you imagine the looks and comments we received seven years ago? Maybe you would see one person a month wearing a mask! Restaurants, large gatherings, Church, and travel were all discouraged. All of us transplants kept containers of hand sanitizer and alcohol wipes in our pockets or purses. So this present situation is familiar to us, except now it has extended to the entire population of the country.

Late July provided the first opportunity to schedule an MRI on that pesky shoulder. The results of the test were disturbing. With a serious rotator cuff tear and a frayed bicep tendon, surgery was planned for the last week of August.

Repair and reconstruction of the shoulder went smoothly. The timing of the surgery seemed fortuitous since the pace of work had become manageable again and the pool remained closed. Recovery actually progressed much slower when compared to the heart transplant. Twice weekly rehab sessions and countless hours of at-home strength building and stretching exercises eventually prepared me for a return to the pool after Thanksgiving.

Eight months out of the pool (the second-longest absence in 55 years), shoulder surgery and recovery, cataract surgery, shingles, working harder than a one-armed bandit in Las Vegas, Covid-19—2020 was one for the record books. Yet, I am thankful for life with its challenges and eternally grateful to my donor and his family's generous gift of life.

2020 is gone, thank God. I got vaccinated for Covid-19, and back in the pool again.

The New Year brought another miracle to our family. On January 10 my wife was given the gift of life by another unknown hero. Jean received a kidney and has done remarkably well. Just a fun fact, as they wheeled Jean into the surgery room, the surgeons showed her the kidney they would soon transplant into her. She remarked after surgery since the kidney was cold it looked like a chicken breast. You can't say one experiences that too often!

It is my hope that this book brings some kind of encouragement to all who read it.

Always in loving memory of my kindred spirit and Transplant Brother, Gordon Veldman,

Fred Nelis (or you can call me by my nickname, Woody Newheart)
Spring, 2021

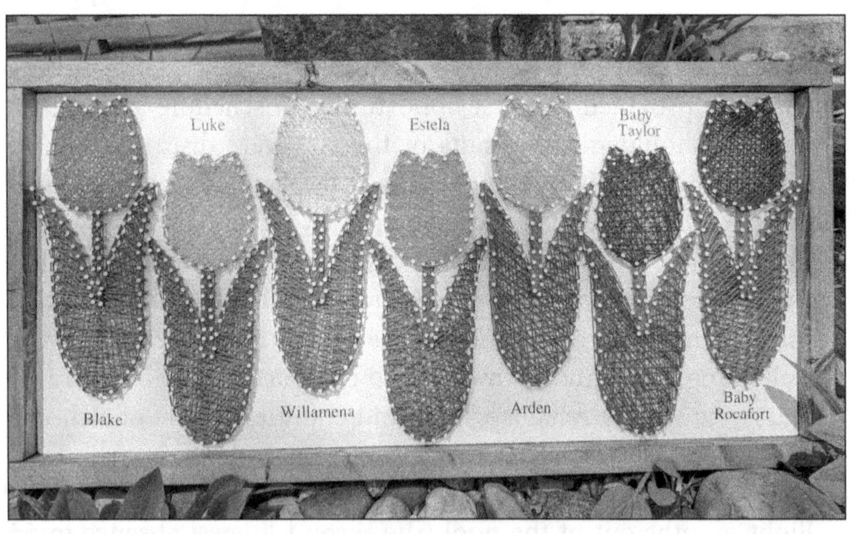

Welcoming two more grandchildren in 2021

Appendix

A BRIEF HISTORY OF ORGAN
TRANSPLANTATION

THIS NARRATIVE has taken for granted the existence of transplant as a medical commonplace. Fred and Gordon, however, never failed to look upon the process as anything less than miraculous. This appreciation and reverence holds true for most transplant recipients and their families, and as transplant becomes more and more a part of the landscape, it is worth pausing to remember just how recently the procedure became a viable medical option.

The historical record is rife with evidence that the prospect of transplantation has fascinated humans for millennia. However, it would take until the late nineteenth and twentieth centuries for the development of the scientific knowledge and surgical techniques that would turn that metaphysical dream into a medical reality.

There are a number of types of transplants: Autotransplantation refers to a transplant (an autograft) from one part of the body to another in the same person, syngeneic transplantation is the term for grafts transplanted between two genetically identical individuals of the same species, such as twins, and xenotransplantation is the grafting or transplanting of organs or tissues between members of different species.

This book is mainly concerned with the concept of allotransplantation, the transfer of cells, tissues, or organs to a recipient from a genetically non-identical donor of the same species, a process that failed for thousands of years due to a lack of understanding of the science surrounding rejection. The transplanted organ is referred to as an allograft, allogeneic transplant, or homograft. Most human tissue and organ transplants, including those of Fred and Gordon, are allografts.

The early mythology of many cultures features miraculous accounts of xenotransplantation performed by gods, priests, and shaman, and of mythical conjoined creatures that resulted from these efforts. In Greek mythology, the Chimera was a destructive, hybrid creature often depicted as part lion, goat, and snake.

Some early texts describe rudimentary autografts, such as skin grafts, considered to be the first organ transplants. Hindu texts dating back as far as 3000 BC depict skin grafts cut from an individual's buttocks, chin, or forehead to reconstruct noses cut off as a punishment for crimes. By 800 BC, Indian physicians had likely mastered skin graft technology as a method to repair burns and wounds.

In the West, the technique was mastered by sixteenth-century Italian surgeon Gasparo Tagliacozzi, sometimes known as the father of plastic surgery. Tagliacozzi reconstructed noses and ears using skin from patients' arms. He found that skin from a different donor usually caused the procedure to fail, observing the immune response that would come to be recognized as transplant rejection.

By the early twentieth century, many European doctors focused attention on trying to save patients dying of renal failure by transplanting kidneys from animals, including monkeys, pigs, and goats. None of the recipients lived for more than a few days. However, over the next several decades, breakthroughs would occur in the successful transplantation of bone, skin, and corneas. In 1905, Eduard Zirm, an Austrian ophthalmologist, performed the world's first corneal transplant, restoring the sight of a man who had been blinded in an accident.

Two breakthroughs with a major impact on later organ transplant success occurred in the pioneering work of the French surgeon, Alexis Carrel, who received the 1912 Nobel Prize for the improvements he developed to suture blood vessels. The technique of "triangulation," using three stay-sutures as traction points to minimize damage to the vascular wall, was inspired by sewing lessons he took from an embroideress and is still used in vascular surgery today. Along with the aviator Charles Lindbergh, he also invented the first perfusion pump, a device for keeping organs viable outside the body and a precursor to the artificial heart, opening the way to modern organ transplantation.

In 1933, the Ukrainian surgeon Yurii Voronoy achieved the first human kidney transplant, using an organ from a deceased donor. The recipient died two days later as a result of rejection. In the late 1940s and early 1950s, doctors at Boston's Peter Bent Brigham Hospital carried out a series of human kidney transplants, some of which functioned for months. In 1954 the surgeons transplanted a kidney from 23-year-old Ronald Herrick into his identical twin brother, Richard, who lived another nine years. Dr. Joseph E. Murray received the Nobel Prize for Medicine in 1990 for this pioneering work.

The next quarter century would see a slew of advancements, including firsts for all the organs commonly transplanted today.

In 1967, after studying with transplant pioneer Dr. Norman Shumway of Stanford University, a young South African heart surgeon, Dr. Christian Barnard, stunned the world by performing the first human heart transplant at Groote Schuur Hospital in Cape Town.

Liver and pancreas transplants were successfully performed by the late 1960s, and lung, combined heart-lung, and intestinal organ transplant procedures began in the 1980s. Two important issues would also be addressed during this time: the definition of brain death and the introduction of immunosuppressive drugs to combat organ rejection.

Technology had improved to the point in the 1960s where the body could be maintained with artificial support long after the brain had died. A new definition of death was required; one that included situations where the entire brain and brain stem had irreversibly ceased to function (brain death). This determination is critical to organ donation as it allows recovery before cessation of blood flow to the organs.

Prior to brain death, organs could only be recovered after the heart had stopped beating, which limited transplants to kidneys and livers only. Brain death allowed the additional recovery of the heart, pancreas, lungs, and intestines. The first standard sets of neurologic criteria for determining death were developed at Harvard University in 1968 and 1969. These criteria have since been adopted by all fifty states, as has the Uniform Anatomical Gift Act that addresses the conditions governing donations.

In 1978, the immunosuppressive drug, Cyclosporin, was introduced and many of the problems of rejection were controlled. The drug received FDA approval for widespread use in 1983. Since then, other drugs have been developed that specifically target only those cells involved in the rejection process while leaving the remaining immune system intact.

In 1984, Congress passed the National Organ Transplant Act, which prohibits the selling of human organs, establishes the Organ Procurement and Transplantation Network (OPTN) to ensure fair and equitable allocation of donated organs, and the Scientific Registry of Transplant Recipients to conduct an ongoing evaluation of the scientific and clinical status of organ transplantation. It also provided for grants for the establishment, initial operation, and expansion of organ procurement organizations.

In 1986, the US Department of Health and Human Services awarded the national OPTN contract to UNOS. UNOS continues as the only organization ever to operate the OPTN. UNOS has established the current organ sharing system, collects and publishes data pertaining to the patient waiting list, organ matching, and transplants, and works to increase the number of organs available for transplantation.

More recent transplant firsts include the first successful living donor liver transplant (1989), first successful living donor lung transplant (1990), first successful hand transplant (1998), first successful partial face transplant (2005), first successful complete full double arm transplant (2008), first baby born from transplanted ovary (2008), first transplant of a human windpipe using a patient's own stem cells (2008), first successful full face transplant (2010), and first double leg transplant (2011). Today, one-year survival rates for most organs are between 70 percent and 90 percent.

DESPITE THESE BREAKTHROUGHS, a common theme continues: that of chronic organ shortages.

At the end of 2019, nearly 114,000 people in the US were on waiting lists for organ transplants; in the prior year, more than 7,000 people on those lists did not live to receive a transplant.

While the number of potential recipients on transplant waiting lists has more than doubled over the past twenty-five years, the number of deceased donors has increased by only half. Meanwhile, the numbers of deaths related to the organ shortage has grown in parallel with the waiting list, continuously increasing the gap between supply and demand.

This ongoing situation has led to the development of a number of suggested approaches, ranging from financial compensation for donors to relaxed standards for donated organs to opt-out programs for donors. Science is also producing new approaches to preserving organs for longer periods of time.

Scientists are revisiting and updating old ideas, including xeno-transplantation and chimeras, and are launching new areas of study, such as regenerative medicine and 3D-printed organs that were undreamed of just a few short years ago.

Researchers at the National Institutes of Health have kept pig hearts beating in the abdomens of baboons for upwards of two years.

The implications for future use in humans are obvious, and the next step is to substitute the pig heart for the baboon heart.

In the world of transplant research, the term, chimera, has taken on the meaning of an entity with multiple genomes. The goal of growing replacement human organs in animals—a controversial idea with numerous technical and ethical impediments—is still a long way from being a practical solution, but it received a jump-start in 2017 with groundbreaking studies published in *Cell* and *Nature.*

In those studies, biologists from the Salk Institute implanted human stem cells into a pig embryo, which contributed to the formation and growth of tissue containing both pig and human cells. And researchers at Stanford and the University of Tokyo reversed diabetes in mice by transplanting mouse pancreas glands that had been grown in a rat.

Scientists are also looking at ways in which damaged organs can potentially heal themselves, negating the need for transplant. Recent studies have shown that the adult human heart generates new muscle cells called cardiomyocytes. The cells are regenerated in sites throughout the heart several times throughout our lives. Uncovering the mechanisms behind cardiomyocyte regeneration could lay the foundation for the development of therapies that harness the heart's regenerative capabilities to heal itself.

In 2018, Johns Hopkins University School of Medicine researchers successfully generated mature heart muscle cells using stem cells. Stem-cell therapy is also at the heart of so-called bio-artificial devices and tissues that are engineered and integrated into a human, to replace or augment a natural organ. Recent breakthroughs include a windpipe made from stem cells that was successfully implanted into a 2-year-old girl in 2012 by scientists from Seoul National University Hospital in South Korea.

The technology of 3D printing has enormous implications for solving the organ shortage problem. In late 2017, surgeons in Australia performed a world-first transplant surgery by successfully implanting a 3D printed tibia wrapped in blood vessels and leg tissue into the leg of a patient facing amputation. The tibia is designed to promote bone growth around it, and slowly dissolve over time.

All these biological and bio-artificial advances are exciting, and many are fraught with ethical considerations. Some experts, however, believe that the solution will not be found in new ways to grow, conserve, and use organs, but in future mechanical and technological breakthroughs such as those that have led to the development of the ventricular assist device (VAD) in recent years. A VAD is an electromechanical device for improving cardiac circulation, used to replace or assist the function of a failing heart. VADs are designed to assist either the right ventricle (RVAD), the left ventricle (LVAD), or both ventricles (BiVAD).

Today, most centers are performing many more VAD surgeries than they are transplant surgeries, and some patients are opting for the quality of life they receive from VADs and other devices in place of transplant.

"In the old days we hardly ever talked to engineers, mathematicians, or biological scientists who were outside of medicine," said Marcus Haw, MD, co-director, Congenital Heart Center, Helen DeVos Children's Hospital and department chief, Pediatric Cardiothoracic Surgery. "Now we interact and collaborate with people from all over the place. It's like crowdsourcing with a lot of clever people in all sorts of institutions.

"Mechanicals are way ahead of a biological solution," he added. "Mechanicals will work in the end."

COEXISTING SIDE-BY-SIDE WITH the science of organ transplant are a number of myths, misconceptions, and unexplained phenomena that have arisen in popular culture.

The popular press, tabloids, and online sites of a wide variety of credibility are loaded with sensationalist stories of organ recipients who mysteriously take on the personality and characteristics or develop the tastes of their donor.

Claire Sylvia, a 47-year-old teacher from Boston and 1988 heart-lung transplant recipient, writes in her memoir, *A Change of Heart*, that she began craving beer and chicken nuggets soon after her transplant surgery, foods she had never enjoyed previously. She also began to have recurring dreams about a man named "Tim L."

A search of the obituaries provided Sylvia with her donor's name and other information. Tim L. was an 18-year-old who died in a motorcycle accident, who also happened to enjoy the foods that she now craved.

These stories are widely reported elsewhere.

A heart transplant recipient named Sonny Graham, of Georgia, married the former wife of his donor. Twelve years after the operation, in 2008, he killed himself with a shotgun—a suicide in the same purported manner as his donor.

Not all these reported incidents are as dramatic as the Sonny Graham case. Many pertain to mundane details such as a change of taste in food or music, or new variations in emotional states.

Dr. Michael Hagan, a Grand Rapids, Michigan, ER physician had a liver transplant after contracting hepatitis C. He says that he experiences new cravings since receiving the transplant more than a decade ago.

"I never ate avocado before; now, I eat an avocado every day," he told WZZM TV-13. "And before my transplant, I never cared for barbecue things, and after my transplant I really liked barbecue."

Something else changed, too, for the veteran ER doctor who was trained to keep his emotions in check.

"After my transplant, I found that I became very, very emotional—so much so that I could go to almost any movie and cry in the movie, and that was very unlike me."

Some theorists turn to the hotly contested theory of cell memory, which holds that memories are stored in the neurons of cells, thus enabling them to live on in the cells of donated organs. Although not widely accepted by academics, this theory has gained several mainstream adherents, most notably Gary Schwartz, PhD, a professor of psychology, medicine, neurology, psychiatry, and surgery at the University of Arizona, his wife, the clinical psychologist Linda

Russek, PhD, and best-selling author and clinical neuropsychologist, the late Paul Pearsall, PhD, of the University of Hawaii.

Several studies applying this hypothesis to organ recipients and additional studies investigating changes in organ recipient personalities have been carried out, although with very small sample sizes and relying primarily on questionnaire and anecdotal evidence.

Schwartz and Russek teamed up with Pearsall for a study published in 2005. The evidence presented is anecdotal, but compelling.

Case 10: The donor was a 34-year-old police officer shot attempting to arrest a drug dealer. The recipient was a 56-year-old college professor diagnosed with atherosclerosis and ischemic heart disease.

The donor's wife reported: '…Casey [the recipient's wife] said offhandedly that the only real side-effect of Ben's surgery was flashes of light in his face. That's exactly how Carl died. The bastard shot him right in the face. The last thing he must have seen is a terrible flash.'

The recipient reported: 'If you promise you won't tell anyone my name, I'll tell you what I've not told any of my doctors. Only my wife knows. I only knew that my donor was a 34-year-old very healthy guy. A few weeks after I got my heart, I began to have dreams. I would see a flash of light right in my face and my face gets real, real hot. It actually burns.'

Cellular memory theory is widely disputed, since the prevailing neurobiological theory has long held that long-term memories are stored at synapses, the junctions between cells, not in the neurons of the cells themselves.

However, a landmark 2014 study by UCLA researchers in the online journal *eLife* suggests that traces of a lost memory might remain in a cell's nucleus, lending possible support to cellular memory theory. Using the neurotransmitter serotonin to trigger synapse growth in neurons, researchers found that when they inhibited this growth with an enzyme, the neuron later "remembered" how many synapses it is supposed to form, meaning it somehow stored this information, challenging the idea that only stable synapses store long-term memories.

And in 2018, UCLA researchers again published a study challenging the prevailing theory. In this case, they transplanted RNA from the nervous system of a snail that had been trained to respond to electrical stimulation. When the material was transplanted into a second group of snails, they demonstrated that they retained a "memory" of the stimulation by overreacting much more strongly to sensory stimulation than a control group of snails.

Other experts, transplant clinicians who work in the field, suggest a more mundane explanation than cellular memory theory for these sensational coincidences in human beings.

"What does happen is the fact that transplantation is obviously a life-transforming and lifesaving procedure," Professor Gurch Randhawa, an organ donation specialist and director of the Institute for Health Research at the University of Bedfordshire told the *Telegraph*. "Clearly when people need a transplant their health and wellbeing is deteriorating. Physically, psychologically, and emotionally they are becoming drained. So, a lot of patients who then receive a transplant will feel energized."

"With other patients you don't talk about patient history," said Asghar Khaghani, MD, former surgical director of the Spectrum Health Richard DeVos Heart and Lung Transplant Program. "But transplantation is different. You've got organs that come from somebody else. You've got these stories that go around. You've got myths that go around.

"Recipients get a lot of second-hand information. People find out about their donors. The immunosuppressive drugs also have a powerful effect. They can change your taste in food or music and even your personality. It's not unusual and not surprising actually."

Because the patient is in a heightened emotional state, Khaghani says he or she clings to the information as a way to connect with the person giving them new life. Even the Schwartz, Russek, Pearsall study acknowledges this more conventional explanation of the "effects of the immunosuppressant drugs, psychosocial stress, and preexisting psychopathology of the recipients."

However, Khaghani and other experts also leave room for doubt.

"These are very difficult things to investigate on a formulaic scientific basis," Professor Peter Friend, Head of Transplantation at Oxford University and a consultant transplant surgeon told the *Telegraph*. "But that is not assuming there is nothing in it. My personal gut feeling is we have no scientific rationale to support this, but we should also be open-minded about things we can't explain."

"Much of this belief is pseudoscience," Khaghani said. "I don't believe in the genetic transfer. But, one cannot be dogmatic about that. Science fiction becomes reality 200 years from now."

A more important, pervasive mythology impacts the way that many prospective donors approach the idea of organ donation and is one factor in the chronic organ shortage.

The US Health and Human Service's Government Information on Organ Donation and Transplantation publishes the following Myths about Organ Donation, which, despite the best efforts of education and advocacy, continue to persist:

MYTH: **I have a medical condition, so I can't be a donor.**
FACT: Anyone, regardless of age or medical history, can sign up to be a donor. The transplant team will determine at an individual's time of death whether donation is possible. There are very few conditions that would prevent a person from becoming a donor—such as HIV infection, active cancer, or a systemic infection. You should still consider registering. Even with an illness, you may be able to donate your organs or tissues.

MYTH: **I'm too old to be a donor.**
FACT: There's no age limit to organ donation. To date, the oldest donor in the US was age 93. What matters is the health and condition of your organs when you die.

MYTH: **I don't think my religion supports donation.**

FACT: Most major religions in the United States support organ donation and consider donation as the final act of love and generosity toward others.

MYTH: **If they see I'm a donor at the hospital, they won't try to save my life.**

FACT: When you are sick or injured and admitted to a hospital, the one and only priority is to save your life. Period. Donation doesn't become a possibility until all lifesaving methods have failed.

MYTH: **Rich or famous people on the waiting list get organs faster.**

FACT: A national computer system matches donated organs to recipients. The factors used in matching include blood type, time spent waiting, other important medical information, how sick the person is, and geographic location. Race, income, and celebrity are NEVER considered.

MYTH: **My family won't be able to have an open casket funeral if I'm a donor.**

FACT: An open casket funeral is usually possible for organ, eye, and tissue donors. Through the entire donation process, the body is treated with care, respect, and dignity.

MYTH: **My family will have to pay for the donation.**

FACT: There is no cost to donors or their families for organ or tissue donation.

MYTH: **Somebody could take my organs and sell them.**

FACT: Federal law prohibits buying and selling organs in the US. Violators can be punished with prison sentences and fines.

MYTH: **If I'm in a coma, they could take my organs.**

FACT: The majority of deceased organ donors are patients who have been declared brain dead. But brain death is NOT the same as coma. People can recover from comas, but not from brain death. Brain death is final.

MYTH: People in the LGBT community can't donate.
FACT: There is no policy or federal regulation that excludes a member of the LGBT community from donating organs. What matters in donating organs is the health of the organs.

While it is interesting to entertain the possibility of genetic transfer, it is more important, for the sake of the nearly 114,000 people in the US on transplant wait lists and their loved ones, that these prevailing misconceptions be addressed.

Bibliography

INTERVIEWS

Bates, Paula. Personal interview. 12 August 2017.

Bates, Ross. Personal interview. 12 August 2017.

Beard, Laurie. Personal interview (telephone). 15 June 2018.

Boeve, Theodore. Personal interview. 28 April 2017; 30 May 2017.

Brady, Sarah. Personal interview (email/telephone). 20 June 2017.

Brooks, Zach. Personal interview (telephone). 4 June 2017.

Busman, Denise. Personal Interview. 2 June 2017.

Caesar, Jill. Personal interview. 28 June 2017.

Crain, Mary Beth. Personal interview. (numerous: 2015–2018).

Davis, Ralph. Personal interview (telephone). 17 March 2018.

Dickinson, Michael. Personal interview. 18 December 2015;
    17 May 2017.

Dykstra, Heather. Personal interview. 29 June 2017.

Fisher, Margo. Personal interview (telephone). 17 March 2018.

Fogarty, Bev. Personal/telephone interviews. 24 September 2017;
    20 December 2017.

Gerlach, Kathie. Personal interview (telephone). 9 June 2017.

Girgis, Reda. Personal interview. 31 May 2018.

Green, Gary. Personal interview (telephone). 1 June 2017.

Grote, Mary. Personal interview (telephone). 15 April 2018.

Hall, Chrissie. Personal interview. 24 September 2017.

Hall, Dave. Personal interview. 24 September 2017.

Haw, Marcus. Personal interview. 13 June 2017.

Jasker, Janet. Personal interview (telephone). 21 January 2018.

Kenjorski, Heide. Personal interview. 12 August 2017.

Kew, Wally. Personal interview. 12 August 2017.

Khaghani, Asghar. Personal interview. 18 December 2015;
    26 May 2017.

Kitsch, Steve. Personal interview (telephone). 16 April 2018.

Kreutz, Andreas. Email interview. 12, 13 March 2018.

Langholz, David. Personal interview. 18 December 2015;
    13 June 2017.

Levine, Benjamin. Personal interview (telephone). 17 August 2018.

Lorenz, Michelle. Personal interview. 18 December 2015.

Nelis, Charlotte. Personal interview. 29 June. 2017.

Nelis, Fred. Personal interview. (numerous: 2015–2018).

Nelis, Jami. Personal interview. 29 June 2017.

Nelis, Jean. Personal interview. (numerous: 2015–2018).

Nelis, Kevin. Personal interview. 10 January 2018.

Nelis, Pat. Personal interview. 10 January 2018.

Nelis, Tom. Personal interview (telephone). 15 April 2018.

Nicholas, Kelly. Personal interview. 29 June 2017.

Olney, Bill. Personal Interview. 11 August 2017.

Olney, Katherine. Personal interview. 11 August 2017.

Rocafort, Lindsey. Personal interview. 29 June 2017.

Ryan, Bill. Personal interview. 29 May 2018.

Shore, Rebecca. Personal interview. 12 June 2017.

Siegers, Dave. Personal interview. 15 February 2018.

Siewert, Barb. Personal interview. 24 September 2017.

Siewert, Greg. Personal interview. 24 September 2017.

Spitler, David. Personal interview (telephone). 17 May 2018.

Stafford, Randall. Personal interview (telephone). 14 June 2017.

Steponski, Ashley. Personal interview. 27 April 2015.

Steponski, Joe. Personal interview. 27 April 2015.

Stillman, Alicia. Personal interview. 27 April 2015.

Stillman, Michael. Personal interview. 27 April 2015.

Steuber, Karen. Personal interview. 28 June 2017.

Vande Bunte, John. Personal interview. 12 August 2017.

Van Wylen, Steve. Personal interview (telephone). 6 March 2018.

Veine, Krista. Personal interview. 12 June 2017.

Veldman, Gordon. Personal interview. (numerous: 2015–2017).

Vogelsang, Kathleen. Personal interview. 2 October 2017.

Werlein, Holly. Personal interview. 1 June 2017.

Wilton, Penny. Personal interview. 4 August 2017.

Zielinski, Nancy. Personal Interview. 23 July 2017; 24 September
2017; 14 November 2017.

PRESS

ABC News Radio. "Friends Get Organ Transplant from Same
Donor." 11 March 2015.

Aleccia, Jonel. "'I could feel his heart:' Organ donor families bond
with recipients after transplants." NBC News. 27 Nov. 2013. Web
17 April 2018.

Associated Press. "2 Suicide Victims Shared Same Heart, Wife."
1 September, 2008. Web 6 December, 2017.

Barnes, John. "Crash injuries claim Forest Hills Eastern student
Rebecca Vogelsang." *The Grand Rapids Press*. 7 March 2008.
MLive. Web. 11 January 2018.

Begnoche, Steve. "Bond grows after friends receive transplants of
heart, lungs from same donor." *Ludington Daily News*. 28 March
2015.

Begnoche, Steve. "Feeling Fabulous: Gordon Veldman." *Ludington
Daily News*. 8 April 2010. Web. 19 December 2017.

Begnoche, Steve. "Sailing into '91." *Ludington Daily News*. 2 January
1991. Page 1.

Begnoche, Steve. "Take time for what's really important." *Ludington Daily News*. 27 June 2017.

Carter, Brody. "Two Friends, One Donor." WXMI TV-17. 9 March 2015.

Crain, Mary Beth. "Larger than life—and death." *Oceana's Herald-Journal*. 28 Sept. 2017.

Crain, Mary Beth. "The transplant brothers." *Oceana's Herald-Journal*. 1 April 2015.

Crain, Mary Beth. "Transplant brothers: Gordon Veldman and Fred Nelis share a remarkable story of a second chance at life." *Pentwater This Week*. 2 June 2015.

Daugherty, Greg. "The Last Adventure of Richard Halliburton, the Forgotten Hero of 1930s America." *Smithsonian.com*. 25 March 2014. Web. 2 June 2018.

Ellison, Garret. "Riot of 1967: As Detroit burned, Grand Rapids experienced its own civil unrest." *The Grand Rapids Press*. 28 April 2015. *MLive.com*. Web. 5 Jan. 2018.

Firger, Jessica. "Two friends become 'transplant brothers.'" *CBS News*. 10 March 2015.

Foucher, Shawn. "Hope floats." *Spectrum Health Beat*. 24 June 2016.

Grinczel, Steve. "Dream-Cruising Holland Pair Caught in Target Practice." *The Grand Rapids Press*. September 1980.

Grinczel, Steve. "Shots puncture 'dream cruise.'" *The Muskegon Chronicle/Booth News Service*. 25 September 1980. Page 10.

Gruber, Sheila. "Sailing adventure was worth the work." *The Holland Sentinel*. Page 1. 30 April 1983.

Harger, Jim. "For Rich DeVos, giving away his millions was a full-time job." *The Grand Rapids Press*. 10 September 2018. *MLive.com*. Web. 7 Oct. 2018.

Harger, Jim. "Mother of organ donor shares touching story for Buddy Day in Michigan." *The Grand Rapids Press*. 6 April 2010. *MLive.com*. Web. 19 Jan. 2018.

Havenga, Marie. "Young at heart." *Spectrum Health Beat*. 10 June 2016.

Hawkins, Tim. "A silver lining." *Spectrum Health Beat*. 8 August 2017.

Hawkins, Tim. "Helping the heart heal itself." *Spectrum Health Beat*. 6 August 2015.

Hawkins, Tim. "Transplant brothers share more than friendship." *Spectrum Health Beat*. 15 April 2015.

Hopkins, Carol. "West Bloomfield family of meningitis victim urges organ donation." 2 September 2013. *Oakland Press*. Web. 17 April 2018.

"Idle shooting wounds boat owner." *The Milwaukee Journal*. 23 September 1980. Page 1.

Jahnke, Pam. "Couple ready for year-long cruise: A dream finally comes true." *The Holland Sentinel*. 13 September 1980. Page 16.

Killian, Chris. "Heartbeat." Kalamazoo College News and Events. Kzoo.edu. 10 March 2014. Web. 17 April 2018.

King, Kyla. "How Rahn Bentley came to be Grand Rapids' first heart transplant patient on Saturday." *The Grand Rapids Press*. 30 Nov. 2010. *MLive.com*. Web. 28 April 2017.

King, Kyla. "Identity of man who donated heart to Grand Rapids' first heart transplant recipient, Rahn Bentley, is revealed." *The Grand Rapids Press*. 6 Dec. 2010. *MLive.com*. Web. 12 June 2017.

King, Kyla. "News that Tim Korzen donated a heart to Grand Rapids' first heart transplant recipient prompts donor list sign ups." *The Grand Rapids Press*. 7 Dec. 2010. *MLive.com*. Web. 12 June 2017.

King, Kyla. "Why Grand Rapids? Q&A with top surgeon hired to lead Spectrum Health's new transplant program." *The Grand Rapids Press*. 8 July 2010. *MLive.com*. Web. 28 April 2017.

Lego, Valerie. "Can organ donations transplant personal qualities?" WZZM TV-13 (reprinted in *Detroit Free Press; Freep.com*). 5 February 2015. Web. 1 December 2017.

Levin, Doron. "Fate, patience bring DeVos a new heart: Amway cofounder back after journey for life." *Detroit Free Press*. 8 Oct. 1997. *Freep.com*. Web. 1 May 2017.

McAvoy, Koco. "Two Friends Receive Organ Donation from Same Donor." WOOD TV-8. 9 March 2015.

"Michigan student's death continues to help save lives of others." *ClickOn Detroit.com.* 12 November 2014. Web. 17 April 2018.

Reens, Nate. "Rahn Bentley's journey from hospital bed to hospitality during Thanksgiving." *MLive.com.* 25 Nov. 2011. Web. 5 May 2017.

Rudavsky, Shari. "'This room becomes sacred.' The heroic and heartbreaking journey of one organ donor's body." *IndyStar.com.* 17 May 2018. Web. 23 May 2018.

"Sailing adventure halted by another adventure." *The Holland Sentinel.* 23 September 1980.

"Sailor won't let bullet scuttle plans for trip." *The Milwaukee Journal.* 25 September 1980.

Samuel, Leah. "To solve organ shortage, states consider 'opt-out' organ donation laws." *STAT.* 6 July 2017. Web. 31 October 2017.

Sanchez, Mark. "Spectrum Health pitches for heart transplant in Grand Rapids." *Business Review West Michigan.* 5 January 2010. Web. 6 June 2017.

Sanchez, Mark. "Spectrum Health seeks state OK to do heart transplants in Grand Rapids." *Business Review West Michigan.* 1 Oct. 2009. Web. 6 June 2017.

Schneider, Keith. "Grand Rapids Lays the Foundation for a Health Mecca." *New York Times.* 11 July 2007. Web. 16 June 2017.

Shute, Joe. "The life-saving operations that change personalities." *Telegraph.* 6 Feb 2015. Web. 31 Oct 2017.

Spectrum Health. Press Release. "Spectrum Health Performs Its First Heart Transplant: 50-Year-Old Grand Rapids Man Receives New Heart Thanksgiving Weekend." *Spectrum Health.* 30 Nov. 2010. Web. 1 May 2017.

Thoms, Sue. "First local heart transplant performed on football star Ray Bentley's brother." *The Grand Rapids Press.* 30 Nov. 2010. *MLive.com.* Web. 5 May 2017.

Thoms, Sue. "Grand Rapids first heart transplant recipient Rahn Bentley announces foundation that will raise scholarship money for donor's sons." *The Grand Rapids Press*. 14 Dec. 2010. *MLive. com*. Web. 5 May 2017.

Thoms, Sue. "Parents share emotional meeting with men who received donor organs from their 19-year-old daughter." *The Grand Rapids Press*. 18 Sept. 2013. *MLive.com*. Web. 17 April 2018.

Thoms, Sue. "Profile: Heart surgeon Dr. Asghar Khaghani." *The Grand Rapids Press*. 18 April 2011. *MLive.com*. Web. 28 April 2017.

Thoms, Sue. "Top heart surgeon explains why he is leaving England to expand Grand Rapids pediatric program." *The Grand Rapids Press*. 31 May 2012. *MLive.com*. Web. 6 June 2017.

Thoms, Sue. "Transplant brothers: Friends receive organs from same donor." *The Grand Rapids Press*. Page A5. 10 March 2015.

Thoms, Sue. "Transplant surgeon becomes middle schoolers' able assistant as class dissects hearts." *The Grand Rapids Press*. 14 Dec. 2013. *MLive.com*. Web. 28 April 2017.

Wein, Harrison. "Long-lived pig-to-primate heart transplants." *NIH Research Matters*. 19 April 2016. Web. 14 October 2018.

Willingham, A. A. "Scientists have transplanted memory from one snail to another. So, what does it mean for humans?" *CNN.com*. 17 May 2018.

Zadorozny, Chis. "Holland's Fred Nelis breaks world record at World Transplant Games." *The Holland Sentinel*. 6 September 201

PEER-REVIEWED JOURNALS

Bédécarrats, Alexia, David L. Glanzman, et al. "RNA from Trained Aplysia Can Induce an Epigenetic Engram for LongTerm Sensitization in Untrained Aplysia." *eNeuro*. 14 May 2018.

Bunzel, B., et al. "Does changing the heart mean changing personality? A retrospective inquiry on 47 heart transplant patients." *Quality of Life Research*. 1992; Vol. 1: 251–6.

Chen, S., et al. "Reinstatement of long-term memory following erasure of its behavioral and synaptic expression in Aplysia." *Elife*. 2014 Nov 17; 3:e03896.

Hippen, Benjamin, Lainie Friedman Ross, and Robert M. Sade. "Saving Lives Is More Important Than Abstract Moral Concerns: Financial Incentives Should Be Used to Increase Organ Donation." *The Annals of Thoracic Surgery*. 88.4 (2009): 1053–1061. PMC. Web. 15 Dec. 2017.

Joshi, S. "Memory transference in organ transplant recipients." *Journal of New Approaches to Medicine and Health*. Volume 19. Issue 1. 24 April 2011.

Pearsall, Paul, et al. "Changes in heart transplant recipients that parallel the personalities of their donors." *Journal of Near-Death Studies*. Spring 2002; 20:3.

Pearsall, Paul, et al. "Organ transplants and cellular memories." *Nexus Magazine*. April/May 2005; 12:3.

Schwartz G., and L. Russek. "The origin of holism and memory in nature: The systemic memory hypothesis." *Frontier Perspectives* .1998; 7(2):23–30.

Schwartz G., and L. Russek. "The plausibility of homeopathy: The systemic memory mechanism." *Integrative Medicine*. 1998; 1(2):53–60.

Skillings, J. L., and Amber Lewandowski. "Team-Based Biopsychosocial Care in Solid Organ Transplantation." *Journal of Clinical Psychology in Medical Settings*. 2015. 22: 113–121.

Watson, C. J. E., and J. H. Dark. "Organ transplantation: historical perspective and current practice." *British Journal of Anaesthesia*. Volume 108, Issue suppl. 1. 1 January 2012. Pages i29–i42.

BOOKS/FILMS

Arlinsky, Ellen, and Marg Ed Kwapil. *In Celebration of Grand Rapids*. Windsor Publications. 1987.

Bentley, Rahn B. *Off to See the Wizard*. Author. 2011.

Calvin, John. *Commentaries on Election and Predestination.*

Daugavietis, Pamela Harman. *The Gift of All: A Community of Givers* (Film). Grand Rapids Community Foundation. 2009.

DeVos, Rich. *Simply Rich: Life and Lessons from the Cofounder of Amway: A Memoir.* Howard/Simon and Schuster. 2016.

Durrett, Deanne. *Organ Transplants.* Lucent Books. 1993.

Elliott, Gerald. *Grand Rapids: Renaissance on the Grand.* Continental Heritage Press. 1982.

Kackley, Rod. *Last Chance Mile: The Reinvention of an American Community.* Abbott Press. 2012.

Lewis, Norma. *Grand Rapids, Furniture City.* Arcadia Publishing. 2008.

Lydens, Z. Z. *The Story of Grand Rapids.* Kregel Publications. 1966.

Massie, Larry B. *A Grand Adventure: The Heritage of Grand Rapids, Michigan.* Heritage. 2001.

Olson, Gordon L. *A Grand Rapids Sampler.* Grand Rapids Historical Commission. 1992.

Olson, Gordon L. *Grand Rapids, A City Renewed: A History Since World War II.* Grand Rapids Historical Commission.1996.

Parr, Elizabeth, and Janet Mize. *Coping with an Organ Transplant.* Avery. 2001.

Petechuk, David. *Organ Transplantation.* Greenwood Press. 2006.

Samuelson, Linda, Andrew Schrier, et al. *Heart & Soul: The Story of Grand Rapids Neighborhoods.* William B. Eerdmans Publishing Company. 2003.

Sylvia, Claire, and William Novak. *A Change of Heart: A Memoir.* Warner Books. 1997.

Van Andel, Jay. *An Enterprising Life.* HarperCollins. 1998.

ORGANIZATION AND GOVERNMENT WEBSITES

"About Us: From the Netherlands to Holland, Michigan." Nelis' Dutch Village. (dutchvillage.com). 15 November 2017.

"Dutch in GR." *Experience Grand Rapids.* 15 December 2017.

"History – About Transplantation." *Organ Procurement and Transplantation Network* (optn.transplant.hrsa.gov). US Department of Health and Human Services. 10 May 2017.

History.com staff. "Organ Transplants: A Brief History." *History. com.* A+E Networks. 21 February 2012. 10 May 2017.

"History." *UNOS* (unos.org). United Network for Organ Sharing. 10 May 2017.

"History of Organ and Tissue Transplant: Medicine and Law." *MTF Biologics* (mtfbiologics.org). MTF Biologics (Formerly known as the Musculoskeletal Transplant Foundation). 10 May 2017.

"How Donation Works: The organ donation process." Gift of Life Michigan. (giftoflifemichigan.org). 15 November 2017.

"OCS™ Heart: Portable Perfusion and Monitoring." *Transmedics. com.* 1 December 2017.

"Organ Donation Myths and Facts." *US Government Information on Organ Donation and Transplantation* (organdonor.gov). Health Resources & Services Administration of the US Department of Health and Human Services. 1 December 2017.

"Timeline of Historical Events and Significant Milestones." *US Government Information on Organ Donation and Transplantation* (organdonor.gov). Health Resources & Services Administration of the US Department of Health and Human Services. 10 May 2017.

Uptodate.com. 12 December 2018.

OTHER

Care Pages. Fred Nelis. 2014.

Heacock, Steven R. Grand Rapids: The Collaborative City. World Leisure Conference Presentation. 12 September 2014.